15-MINUTE HIIT
FOR WOMEN

15-Minute

HIIT

FOR WOMEN

High-Intensity Workouts You Can Do Anywhere

Gina Harney
Illustrations by Conor Buckley

ROCKRIDGE PRESS

This book is dedicated to my favorite source of never-ending cardio, Olivia and Penelope.

Interior and Cover Designer: Mando Daniel

Art Producer: Sue Bischofberger

Editor: Andrea Leptinsky and Nicky Montalvo

Production Manager: Michael Kay

Production Editor: Melissa Edeburn

Illustration © 2020 Conor Buckley

Photography © Jacob Lund/shutterstock, p. viii; vgajic/iStock, p. 14; oneinchpunch/shutterstock, p. 58; ANRproduction/iStock, p. 82; mihailomilovanovic/iStock, p. 103; Olena Yakobchuk/shutterstock, p. 113; PeopleImages/iStock, p.129; and FatCamera/iStock, p. 134. Author photo courtesy of Kristi Harris Photography.

ISBN: Print 978-1-64611-794-9 | eBook 978-1-64611-795-6

R0

Contents

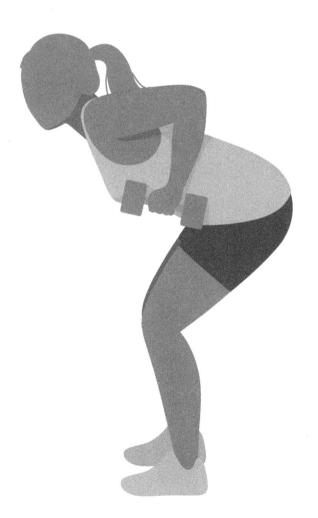

Introduction

HIIT, or high-intensity interval training, has recently become a buzzword in the fitness community. If you've heard of it, challenging exercises like burpees and sprints might come to mind. But HIIT doesn't mean you have to pound your joints or spend half the morning at the gym on complex machines. This book teaches you how to safely and effectively implement a HIIT routine that fits in with your busy lifestyle.

At its most basic level, HIIT consists of periods of hard work followed by periods of rest. This method of training has been scientifically proven to improve heart health, boost fitness performance, and increase metabolism. HIIT workouts are designed to get your heart rate up very quickly, so they'll often consist of plyometric-style exercises (exercises involving power-based dynamic movements like jumping jacks) and calisthenics. A burpee or set of jumping jacks, for instance, will quickly elevate your heart rate—a biceps curl will not.

Some notes about HIIT training:

- During a HIIT interval, you're working at 80 to 95 percent of your max heart rate. If you're using perceived exertion, which is essentially how hard you feel like your body is working, aim for a 9 on a scale of 1 to 10. You should be able to blurt out a couple of words if asked a question, but not be able to speak in full sentences.

- You can use any mode of exercise equipment for HIIT. Rowing machines, spin bikes, stair climbers, battle ropes, and treadmills are all great options. Best are those that are convenient for you.

- HIIT workouts are short! This book is based on 15-minute workouts.

HIIT is a strategic way to train—it gives you more bang for your workout buck. It's like regular cardio, but it's more effective in achieving your overall fitness goals. HIIT may help you lose body fat, but, more significantly, it can also dramatically increase your energy level, help your body fight disease, and improve your life-long health.

I've been a personal trainer and fitness professional for 10 years and have had the honor of working with women at all stages of life. They all shared one constraint: **They didn't have multiple hours a day to try to meet their fitness goals.**

During my last year at the University of Arizona, I fully realized the benefits of fitness and nutrition. I was a finance major, and I often found myself feeling lethargic. So I embarked on a total lifestyle change. I began incorporating whole grains, lean proteins, and fresh produce into my diet. Then I started maximizing my limited time in the gym. On my journey to becoming a personal trainer, I discovered all you need is a smart plan and the motivation to go after your goals.

Why This Book?

With so much HIIT information available, it's hard to know which sources to trust—and it takes precious time to identify them. This book is designed to be your go-to HIIT resource.

This book will set beginners up for success with:

- The definitive guide to proper form and numbers of reps/sets

- Workouts that target major muscle groups as well as the total body, along with strength training

- A resource to keep exercise top-of-mind (when you see it, you achieve it) and track your progress so you can continue to set goals and avoid plateaus

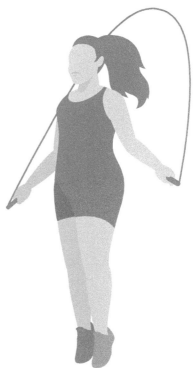

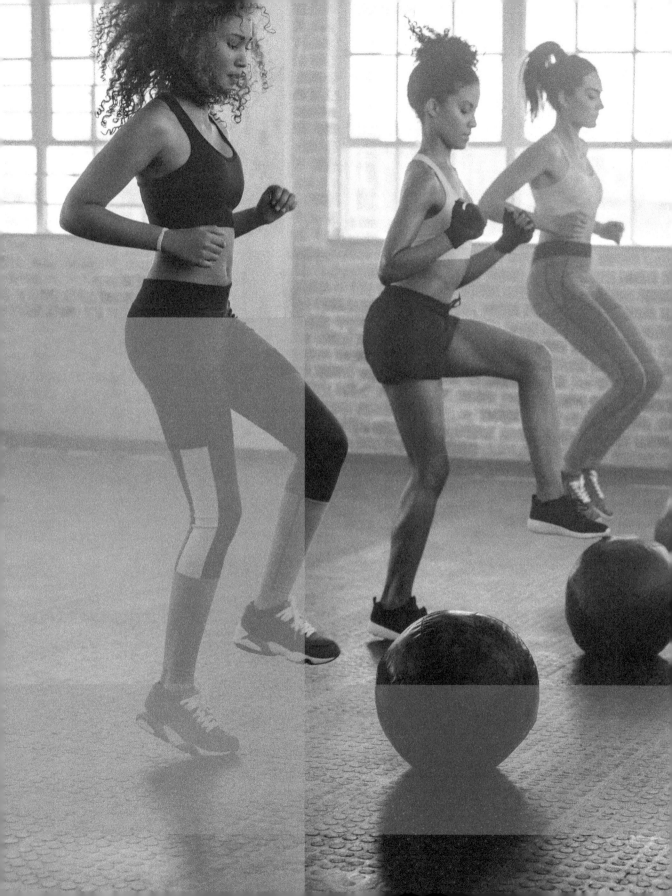

CHAPTER ONE

Understanding High-Intensity Interval Training

I used to feel like any workout less than an hour wasn't worth it, which discouraged me from being active on days I didn't have a huge chunk of time to dedicate to exercise. Years of research and working in the fitness industry have taught me the benefits of HIIT training, but it wasn't until I had my first daughter that I really embraced the beauty of short, effective workouts. I saw incredible results from my post-birth workouts in a third of the time I'd spent on exercise before I became a parent!

You can absolutely get the benefits of a full workout in just 15 minutes with strategic training.

Many people are looking for that magical balance between time and energy: **HIIT is that magical balance.** By incorporating 15-minute HIIT workouts into your routine, you can increase strength, power, stamina, and metabolism while promoting heart health.

Here are some ways women can benefit from HIIT training:

- Increase fat- and calorie-burn

- Lose weight and fat while protecting muscle density

- Improve muscle tone and strength

- Improve bone health

- Improve heart health and cardiometabolic health

Intangible benefits include a reduction in food cravings and improvements in sleep quality and mood.

This book presents goal-setting strategies and an action plan. It answers some common questions (such as when to increase the intensity of workouts) and discusses nutrition's impact on fitness results. Finally, this book lays out HIIT training plans, segmented by major muscle groups.

Everything you need to know to implement the results-proven strategies of HIIT training can be found in this book. All you need is a little motivation and a timer, and you can crush your goals.

Let's HIIT it!

Hows of HIIT

We know that HIIT can be a secret weapon when it comes to effective training, but how does it work?

When we train using HIIT intervals, our bodies have to work hard to quickly increase our heart rate. Then they must work hard to achieve our normal homeostasis (our normal resting state). We consume more oxygen and burn more calories after HIIT workouts than before them.

The remaining portion of the equation is critical. A workout that does not incorporate a break between exercises—say, between burpees and push-ups—is not a HIIT workout. You need time to rest so your heart rate can decrease between rounds.

Here's a more detailed look at how HIIT can affect metabolism, cardiovascular fitness, muscle fiber strength, bone density, and longevity.

METABOLISM

HIIT exercises have positive physiological effects on the ways our bodies turn what we eat and drink into energy. This type of training aids in regulating metabolism by increasing the size and density of the mitochondria (the little fat-burning firehouses in our cells). Additionally, after HIIT, our bodies still work hard to regulate heart rate and lower tissue temperature. We consume more oxygen, a phenomon called excess post-exercise oxygen consumption (EPOC), which increases calorie-burn and helps us reap the benefits of our interval training for the rest of the day.

Because HIIT exercises are anaerobic, our lean muscles are preserved while we're burning calories. HIIT enables us to lose fat while preserving and building muscle tissue, which can boost our metabolism as we age. Muscle is "hungrier" than fat and burns more calories at rest, so the more muscle we can maintain on our frame, the better.

CARDIOVASCULAR FITNESS

A 2010 study showed that HIIT workouts can improve cardiovascular fitness (VO_2max) from 4 percent to 46 percent. Because HIIT exercises increase stroke volume (the amount of blood pumped by the left ventricle of your heart), they deliver more oxygen to the muscles with each pump of the heart. This type of training also increases aerobic endurance, lowers insulin resistance, and increases the density of the aforementioned mitochondria, which positively impacts our ability to handle intense workouts.

MUSCLE FIBER STRENGTH

HIIT focuses on fast-twitch muscle fibers that enable us to complete short and powerful bursts of movement, such as sprinting or jumping. These types of muscle fibers are also "hungrier" than our slow-twitch muscle fibers (those used for long endurance workouts like distance running) and require more fuel. By changing the muscle fibers you're using, you can increase your strength and endurance in comparatively little time. In one 2019 study, participants in both endurance and HIIT groups experienced similar results, but the HIIT group worked out for far less time.

BONE DENSITY

With age, we are more susceptible to bone loss. Resistance training and plyometric-based exercises that focus on maximum muscle force in small amounts of time—like the ones we use in HIIT—put pressure on the bones that can improve overall bone strength. This strength, in turn, can help reduce our chances of developing osteopenia and osteoporosis.

Over time, we are more at risk of losing our independence due to sarcopenia (loss of muscle mass and strength) and overall frailty. In a 2018 study comparing two groups of aging and sedentary mice, the group that completed 10-minute uphill HIIT workouts three times per week for 16 weeks had dramatic improvement in grip strength, treadmill endurance, and gait speed, while they also experienced an increase in muscle fiber mass and strength. Some of these mice became "less frail" and four were ultimately considered non-frail. This finding is a great reminder that it's never too late to make a positive change for your health.

LONGEVITY

HIIT can lower insulin resistance and cholesterol levels because fast-twitch muscles use glucose for fuel. Consequently, glucose levels in the blood drop. Short bursts of exercise can help women who are at risk of developing type 2 diabetes in particular.

Personal Goals

Before you get started, write down some goals.

What do you want to accomplish? How do you want to *feel*? Planning can ensure the consistency needed to maintain a healthy and fit lifestyle—and, ultimately, to achieve the results you want to see.

For many, vanity alone can be a carrot. But will looking good motivate you when you're tired at the end of a long workday? Perhaps a variety of exercises is enticing. But will this variety keep you going long term? You need a goal that will motivate you when you hit a plateau or miss your workout for more than a few days. My goal is to not only look good and feel great now, but also to be a strong woman decades from now so I can garden and chase my grandkids around the park. Find something that motivates *you*.

Put your written goals and motivations in a highly visible place. Each time you see them, you'll be more likely to take small steps each day to achieve what you set out to do. Write your goals as if you will accomplish them—"I will" is more powerful than "I want to." If you like to meditate, spend a couple of minutes each day thinking about your goals and visualizing yourself when you've achieved them. Feel that warmth and excitement in your soul, and use that energy to keep up the hard work.

Remember that goals should be SMART: **S**pecific, **M**easurable, **A**ttainable, **R**ealistic, and **T**imely:

- **Specific:** Translate the general—for example, "I will run faster"—into the specific—"I will run a 10-minute mile."

- **Measurable:** Choose a goal that you can measure, such as, "I will work out at least three times each week," not "I will work out more."

- **Attainable:** Pick a goal that is attainable for you. Once you achieve it, you can push yourself to the next level with a new SMART goal.

- **Realistic:** Consider your time or personal restraints, including lack of enjoyment. If you hate yoga, it's not realistic to say, "I'm going to practice yoga every day."

- **Timely:** Does it make sense for you right now? Is there a deadline you can set for yourself? Give yourself stepping stones to hit at specific intervals (in three months, in six months, in one year) so you can check on your progress.

BEYOND THE BODY

HIIT provides more than incredible physical and physiological benefits. It can improve overall mood and well-being by boosting endorphins and other feel-good hormones, including oxytocin and serotonin. It can impact cognitive performance by boosting cerebral blood flow. When we perform HIIT-style workouts, we're more likely to experience better quality sleep and a reduction in sleep apnea. Just note that it's not a good idea to do a HIIT workout within an hour of bedtime. Researchers have found that those who exercised close to bedtime took 14 minutes longer to fall asleep. Instead, HIIT is a great way to start the day or get a mid-day energy boost.

HIIT Training

How do you know when to start HIIT training?

HIIT is a relatively advanced training technique, but beginners can enjoy its benefits. That said, talk to a doctor before making any fitness or nutrition changes, and honor your body. Don't be afraid to modify exercises according to your body's needs.

Before you jump into a HIIT-style workout, establish a cardio baseline. Make sure you can easily complete 30 minutes of steady-state moderate exercise (like light swimming, walking, jogging, or spinning) most days of the week. At that point, try adding a 30-second speed increase (such as power walking or light running) every five minutes. Once that increase feels good, add a 30-second speed increase every two minutes. Finally, try one minute of walking with a 30-second speed increase. When that increase feels comfortable, you should be ready to complete the HIIT workouts in this book.

If you're new to a consistent fitness regimen, your excitement about doing something great for yourself can sometimes lead to overdoing it. Recovery days are critical in any fitness program, and they're even more necessary if the activity is new to you. Listen to your body and follow your doctor's advice to ensure you mitigate the risk of injury.

If it's your first time performing HIIT exercises, study this book's pictures and form cues. (Bonus points if you meet with a personal trainer who can make sure you're using proper form!) It's much better to execute with proper form and work slowly than it is to risk injury by working too quickly. Use the modified option until it feels manageable for the entire round (30 seconds on and 1 minute off), then try the more advanced version.

Do you increase intensity on the basis of muscle fatigue or heart rate?
Gauge activity by perceived exertion. The work rounds should feel challenging, like an 8 or 9 on a scale of 1 (napping) to 10 (a full-out sprint). As your endurance increases, you may find it necessary to add more advanced variations or to increase speed, resistance, or both to feel that same intensity (if so, congrats on raising your fitness level!). A quick bodyweight squat (page 44) might feel like an 8 or 9 at first but like a 5 or 6 after 4 to 6 weeks of training. If so, you're ready to progress to jump squats, the more advanced version of the exercise.

If you're using a heart rate monitor, HIIT rounds should be 80 to 95 percent of your max heart rate. A simple way to calculate your max heart rate is to subtract your age from 220. So, if you're 35 years old, 220 minus 35 equals 185. The target zones would be 0.80 multiplied by 185 (148) and 0.95 multiplied by 185 (175). In this example, ideally, your heart rate should be anywhere from 148 to 175 beats per minute during your HIIT rounds.

Nutrition

Think of your body like a car. If you fuel your high-performance engine with low-octane, dirty fuel, it's not going to run optimally. Nutrition is an integral factor in health and fitness. Exercise and good nutrition habits work in tandem to support our immune and hormone systems and to help us perform better and achieve our health goals. The meal ideas, fueling strategies, and techniques in this book have worked for me and many of my personal training and weight-loss clients—but I'm not a registered dietitian. If you need help creating a custom meal plan for your personal goals, consider meeting with a registered dietitian in your area.

WHOLE FOODS, NOT FAD DIETS

Fad diets will always exist, and you'll often see social media flooded with recipes focused on the latest dieting trend. Here's the thing: If it seems too good to be true, it probably is. Also, if a diet plan focuses on eliminating entire food groups, it will not be sustainable for the long haul. Once you go back to eating the way you did before the diet, any lost weight will be gained back. (For instance, low-carb diets often result in quick weight loss, but most of that is water weight. Start eating carbs again, and—boom!—it comes back.) Also, any diet that doesn't allow a slice of birthday cake or a glass of wine at dinner isn't a friend of mine. Deprivation diets aren't usually sustainable. You should be able to enjoy foods you love if they're incorporated in a reasonable manner.

Instead of eliminating food groups, focus on eating whole foods rather than heavily processed options. Fresh or frozen fruits and vegetables, nuts, seeds, legumes, whole grains, lean proteins, eggs, dairy (if you enjoy it), and starchy vegetables all have a place on a healthy eating plate. Try to include protein and produce with every meal and snack, and get into the habit of reading ingredient labels. If you don't know what an ingredient is, your body probably won't either.

MODERATION VS. DEPRIVATION

What makes something even more desirable? Telling yourself you can't have it.

Have you ever denied yourself a brownie only to finally give in and eat three or four instead? Deprivation throws portion control out of whack.

Try to get in touch with your cravings and enjoy the foods you love within your healthy eating plan. While I love healthy foods like big salads, veggie burgers, fish, bowls of fruit, and homemade trail mix, I also love less healthy goodies like cake with buttercream frosting, wine, and pizza. So, I allow myself all of these things—in *moderation*. Focusing as much as possible on whole foods can help you feel more satisfied with realistic portions of treats and desserts.

Here's another way to look at it: Think like an athlete. Eat for optimal performance. And if you're following a training plan, you're an athlete, too! Pay attention to how you feel after eating. Which food energizes you? Which makes you feel like you need a nap? Which satisfies you? Try to reduce meals too high in fat, sugar, or starches, because these foods often will make you feel tired and sluggish. Instead, try to eat more foods proven to give the human body extra energy, such as:

- Beans and legumes
- Dairy (Greek yogurt with no added sugar, cottage cheese, milk, etc.)
- Fresh or frozen fruits
- Fresh or frozen vegetables
- Nuts and seeds*
- Nut butters*
- Lean proteins (including chicken, turkey, eggs, fish)
- Starchy vegetables
- Whole grains (like whole-grain pasta, bread)*

*Stay mindful of portion control.

Find staple recipes and ingredients you love and make healthy eating even easier by planning meals in advance.

BREAKFAST

We've all heard that breakfast is important, but it's particularly so when you're exercising in the morning. A good breakfast provides a lot of the nutrients and energy needed to get the most out of your workouts. One of my favorite healthy and delicious morning meals is oatmeal with berries and almond butter. I also love a good egg burrito in a whole-grain tortilla with salsa and grilled or sautéed veggies for protein and vitamins. A smoothie with protein powder gives your body a good boost—I really like one that incorporates frozen berries, almond milk, and chia seeds or chia pudding (simply, 2 tablespoons of chia seeds and 1 cup of almond milk, stirred together and left to set in the fridge overnight) blended with a little honey.

LUNCH

Lunch is a perfect time for incorporating energy-boosting foods that help conquer that mid-afternoon circadian slump that seems to hit around 2:00 p.m. I like savory chickpea curry salad with whole-grain crackers or chicken tacos with shredded lettuce, guacamole, bell peppers, and salsa. On a cold day, I love a good, light soup with a fresh veggie salad (sometimes I add grilled chicken for extra protein). A sandwich packed with veggies or a simple snack of turkey and avocado slices can make eating healthy on the go easy.

DINNER

The last meal of the day should be packed with mouthwatering whole foods that fill you without making you feel stuffed (which can lead to grabbing a bunch of sugary snack foods before bed). Smart choices include a sushi roll bowl (cooked white rice with salmon, cucumber, avocado, nori strips, and sriracha), barbecue chicken with sweet potato and roasted green beans, or roasted chicken with a fresh veggie salad. On the lighter side, you could choose a Cobb salad with romaine, hard-boiled egg, turkey bacon, olives, and feta—just don't forget to inspect the salad dressing's ingredients before eating.

SNACKS

Sometimes we get busy with life and our "three squares" come a little later than we intended. That's okay. Fight the urge to grab an unhealthy snack just because it's handy and sounds good, and opt to eat something your body really needs. A little snacking can help keep your metabolism running, which helps with good choices at mealtime. The key is advanced planning. When you can, plan your snacks and take them with you to work, the park, or for a meet-up with friends. Some snacks that do the trick for me are veggies with hummus, an apple with almond butter, or a small smoothie with almond milk, protein powder, and frozen berries. If you have a couple of extra minutes, try some avocado toast sprinkled with hemp seeds for a truly satisfying mini meal.

SWEETS

Everybody gets the occasional sweet tooth, and it's okay to indulge in moderation. However, you can have a little sweet treat without downing a slice of chocolate cake every time. Instead, try medjool dates with almond butter, a spoonful of peanut butter with chocolate chips, or a simple make-at-home banana "ice cream" (blend a frozen chopped banana in the food processor until it resembles ice cream). Find the healthy treats that gratify your sweet tooth—you'll be surprised how satisfying they can be—all while keeping you on track to achieve your fitness goals.

WORKOUT FUEL

Fueling our workouts provides our bodies with the energy to make the most of them and optimizes muscle recovery. Here are some simple guidelines for what to look for in pre- and post-workout foods.

PRE-WORKOUT

The benefits of doing cardio exercises while fasting, known as fasted cardio, has been well established. In the morning when your body is not using carbohydrates for energy (you've been sleeping, so they've already been burned), fasted cardio can kick you into a fat-burning state more quickly.

But not everyone can work out on an empty stomach. If you need pre-workout fuel, try something small that digests quickly, like a banana with a little peanut butter, a piece of toast, or fruit. If you're working out later in the day, have a satisfying meal or snack an hour or so before your workout to help minimize digestive issues while you exercise.

POST-WORKOUT

You do not need to eat a huge meal after your workout. After strength training, try, instead, a combination of quality proteins, carbs, and a little bit of fat (like a piece of toast with turkey, hummus, and veggies or a smoothie with berries, almond milk, protein powder, and a little peanut butter).

It's a myth that you need to eat within 60 minutes after your workout for optimal results, though with a fasted workout, you'll absolutely need some fuel after you're done. Just ensure you get enough protein, healthy carbs, and smart fats throughout the day. Protein, in particular, is important for preserving lean muscle while you're training.

FAT LOSS

A good rule of thumb for fat loss is to eat like a PRO: Focus on **PRO**tein and **PRO**duce in every meal and snack. To lose the fat, you will need to be in a calorie deficit, but be sure you're eating enough to both fuel your workouts and make your hormones happy. Try filling half your plate with fresh veggies, one quarter with lean protein, and one quarter with a mix of whole grains and healthy fats.

Healthy eating is about more than food, however. Hydration is essential to replace what we sweat out during exercise, and can also promote healthy skin, hair, digestion, and hunger levels. Often, feelings of hunger are magnified

because of dehyrdation. National Academy of Sports Medicine Guidelines sug-
gest we consume at least 96 ounces of water per day, and even more if you're
active. Make your water bottle your BFF.

TIPS FOR GROCERY SHOPPING SUCCESS

- Don't shop while you're hungry. Hunger can lead to impulse buys and options that don't align with your goals.

- Peruse the perimeter first. The good stuff (produce, meat, dairy) hangs out along the outer edges of the store. Then, move to the aisles for nuts and seeds, oatmeal, coffee, tea, and snacks (like jerky, dried fruit, and bars with simple ingredients).

- Check out the bulk bins. Try out new products without having to commit to a huge package while saving on cost.

- Start meal planning. Take time to write down dinners for the week, plus breakfast staples and lunches to enjoy. Create your grocery list from your plan. Food shopping will be faster, you'll avoid impulse buys, and you'll make good use of everything in your well-stocked fridge.

HIIT Anywhere

One of the advantages of HIIT is you can do it anywhere. You don't need a gym membership or access to a lot of fancy equipment. The workouts can be accomplished using only your own body weight and a little motivation. (You can add a set of dumbbells for resistance if you'd prefer an added challenge.) This convenience is especially appealing to those of us who may not have time to drive back and forth to a fitness facility or who may not have the disposable income to pay for expensive gym memberships.

I used to think I couldn't work out unless I went to the gym, but after I had my first daughter, I realized I needed to be able to work out at home to fit it into my schedule. Though both of my kids are in school now, I still gravitate toward home workouts where I can just put on a pair of athletic shoes and get it done!

The exercises in this book are basic and easy to do in various places. You can do them at home, in your office, in the backyard, or while watching the kiddos play. (In my experience, these workouts involve such fun and explosive movements the kids often want to join in!) With just a little bit of space, you'll find that a water bottle, comfortable clothes, and practical shoes are the only tools you need to start an effective fitness journey.

EQUIPMENT

Though you really just need your own body weight for a solid HIIT workout, weights, such as dumbbells, can step up your game. If you don't have dumbbells or other weights, feel free to improvise. A weighted backpack makes a wonderful stand-in for a kettlebell, and a full water bottle can serve as a handheld weight in a pinch. Resistance bands also provide a cheap—and portable—means of taking your exercise session to the next level.

I keep the following items handy:

- Sneakers. Wear comfortable athletic shoes that fit you well.

- Water bottle. Replenish lost water through your workouts. Hydration is essential for optimal cell function, healthy skin, and digestion.

- Weights. I like to use dumbbells, but, as I indicated above, anything weighted will work. For beginners, start with 3- to 5-pound weights for the exercises in this book, then add more weight, as needed. You want a weight that will challenge you but won't feel impossible.

- Resistance bands. Varying degrees of tension allow you to modify exercises to your ability level, and multiple sizes help target different body parts.

- Yoga mat (optional). Some people like to have a cushion for floor work and to help reduce impact on the joints when standing.

- Heart rate monitor (optional). This monitor can be helpful when you're starting to learn your HIIT training zones. (You'll want to be at 80 to 95 percent of your max heart rate for your cardio intervals; refer to page 6 to review the formula for determining this rate.) If you don't have a heart rate monitor, no sweat (pun intended)—gauge your workouts by perceived exertion instead. Simply pay attention to how you feel during the work and recovery rounds. Your work rounds should feel extremely challenging—you should be able to say your address, for example, but not much more—and during your recovery rounds, you should feel your heart rate decrease as your breathing becomes fuller and steadier.

If you'd like to include additional cardio, getting outside for a run has immense value, but even consistently walking can do wonders to improve overall health. Swimming is another healthy option. If it's not practical to be outside, consider jumping rope. Other great sources of cardio include using a treadmill, spin bike, stair climber, or similar machine.

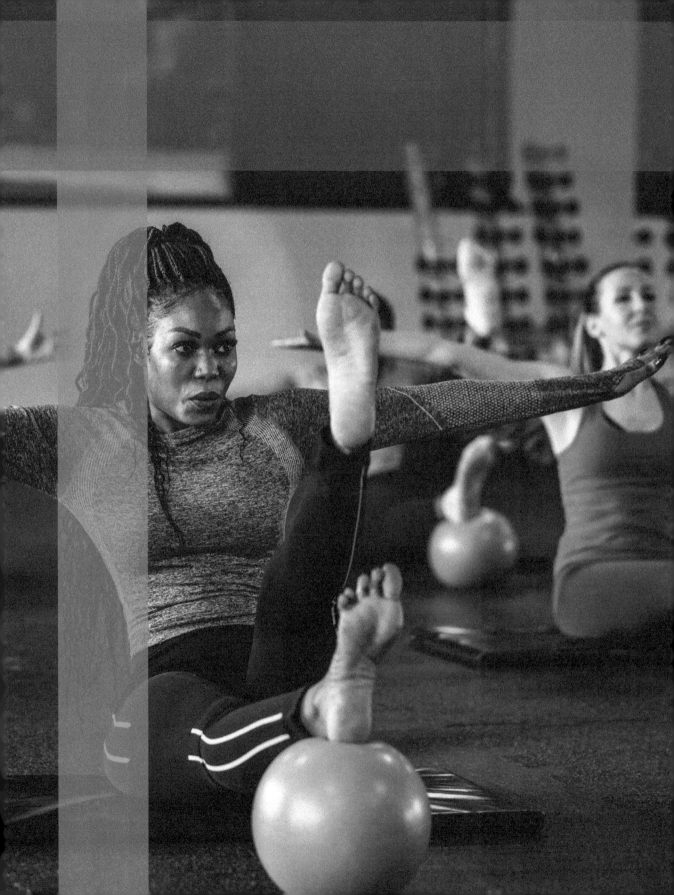

CHAPTER TWO

The Fundamentals

This chapter provides descriptions and illustrated instructions for the basic exercises within the workouts in chapter 3. Warm-up and cool-down exercises are included to help you avoid injury. Consider practicing each exercise before doing your HIIT workout, and be sure to refer to these pages until you master the moves.

Warm-ups

The way you warm-up can either hinder or enhance your performance and is a crucial component of working out. It also helps prevent injuries because you're not going into your workout "cold." Here's an easy way to remember: active stretching (actions mimicking the exercise movements you'll be doing) before you get active, static stretching (holding a position to stretch the muscle) after. For instance, before a workout with jump squats (pages 34, 38, and 44), warm up with bodyweight squats (page 44). During static stretching, you should feel slight pressure but *not* pain. (See the Cool Down section on pages 56–57 for more details.)

More reasons to warm up before exercising:

- Increase circulation and blood flow to the muscles.

- Prepare your body by working safely and slowly through the range of motions you'll be doing.

- Mentally get in the zone before you work out.

My favorite warm-up strategies include:

- Low-to-moderate cardio for 5 to 7 minutes. For example, you might hop on a treadmill, walk around the block, or jump rope for 5 minutes (taking breaks when needed).

- A quick functional circuit. Spend one minute each doing the following exercises: alternating lunge (page 17), jump rope (or jog in place; page 27), plank (page 31), push-up (page 35), and bodyweight squat (page 44).

Throughout this book, I emphasize functional HIIT training—that is, exercises that mimic the way we move during many daily tasks. Many exercises include a quick functional circuit as a warm-up. In other words, perform the workout quickly without adding resistance, almost like a practice run.

Foundational Exercises

This section provides step-by-step instructions for each exercise within the workouts. Each exercise was chosen with time, effectiveness, and safety in mind. Many of the exercises are compound exercises that simultaneously work multiple muscle groups to maximize your results. Others are functional exercises that mimic movements required for squatting, rotating, deadlifting, and planking.

Alternating Lunge

1. Take one very large step forward, keeping your feet in line with your hips. Try to keep your torso perpendicular to the floor as you sink into your lunge.

2. Keep the front knee stacked above the front ankle. As you come up from the lunge, actively think about trying to squeeze your legs together like a pair of scissors.

3. Repeat on the other side.

> **TIP** For Lunge to Pause, complete a standard lunge, stepping forward with one foot and bending both knees 90 degrees. Hold this position for two deep breaths before stepping back into position.

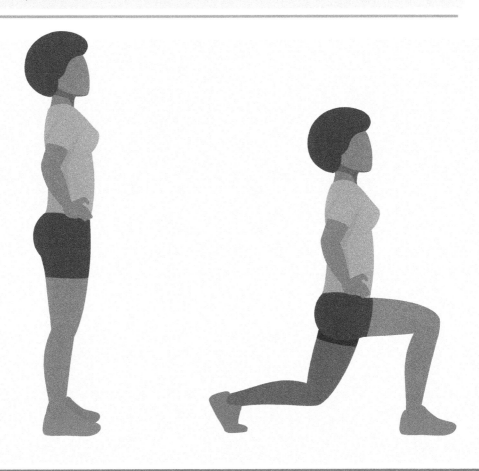

Bent-Over Row

1. Place your feet just under your hips with a slight bend at the knees. Hinge forward from your hips, keeping your back flat (shoulders pulled back) and core tight.

2. Holding a dumbbell (or barbell) in each hand, raise your arms away from the floor, lifting from the rear deltoids and keeping your elbows high and wide.

3. Stop when your arms reach shoulder height before carefully lowering them back down.

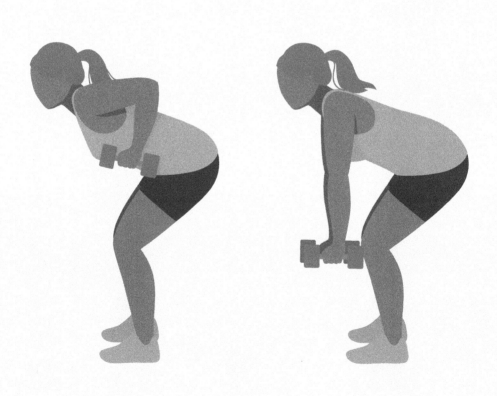

Biceps Curl

1. Keep your elbows close to your torso, maintaining a tight core and a slight bend in your knees. Hold a pair of dumbbells or something you can use for resistance.

2. Lift up through your chest as you flex at the elbow, bringing the weight all the way up (aiming toward your shoulder). As you release, try to resist the weight and go for a nice full extension at the bottom of the movement.

> **TIP** For a Biceps Curl Pulse, hold the weights at a 90-degree angle and make small, repeated, two-inch movements up and down.

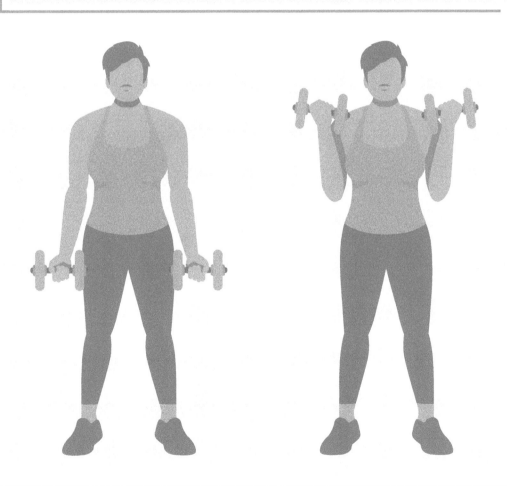

Breakdancer

1. Start on all fours with your hands under your shoulders and knees under your hips.

2. Use the strength of your core to lift your knees off the ground so you're now on your toes.

3. Pivot on your left foot as you bring your right foot through the center to the opposite side. Place your left hand on your head.

4. Come back to all fours and repeat on the opposite side.

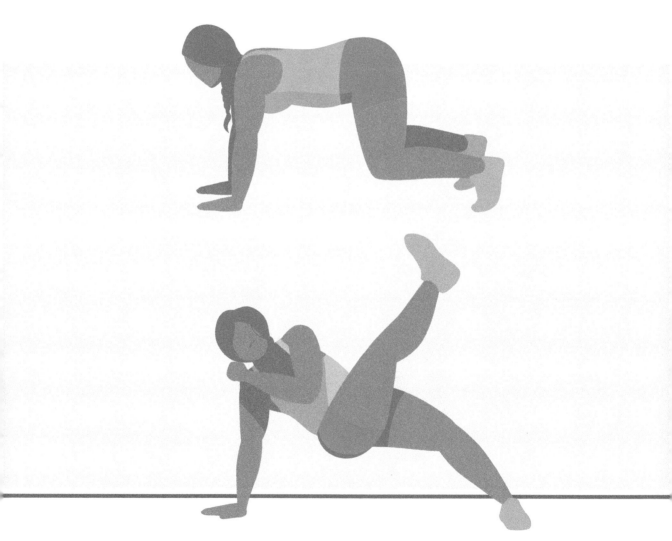

Burpee

1. Squat with flat feet and place both hands on the floor, firmly planting your entire hand.

2. Walk or hop your feet backward into a plank position (a push-up here is optional), then walk or hop your feet back to your hands and jump vertically, raising your arms overhead.

TIP To reduce impact, eliminate the jump. To reduce core pressure, place your hands on a wall or a sturdy bench.

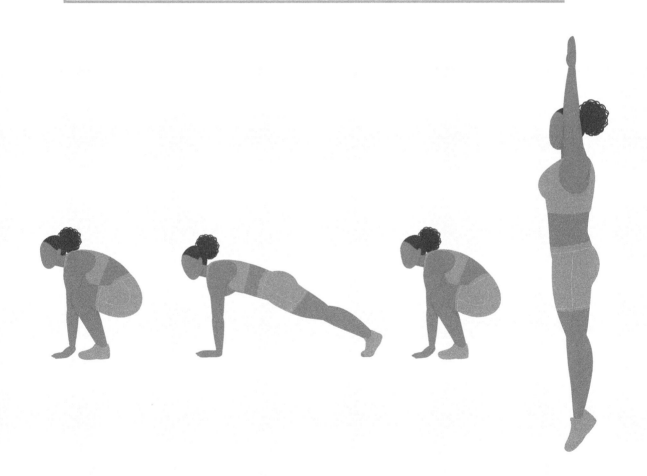

Close Squat

1. Stand with your feet and legs close together.

2. Begin to move toward a squatting position, sitting back while keeping your chest lifted and core tight.

3. Inhale to lower, exhale to rise. Make sure your knees extend toward, but not past, your toes.

4. Sink your hips as low as your flexibility allows, whether it's a small squat or just above knee level.

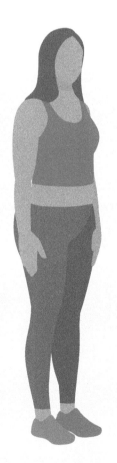
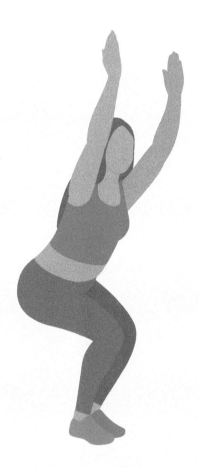

Cobra

1. Lie down on your stomach. Stretch your body out with your head facing down. Your torso, thighs, and feet should be firmly planted on the floor.

2. Lift your legs and torso by extending your hips and spine. Raise your arms simultaneously, palms facing upward. Maintain the position for as long as you can.

3. Lower with control.

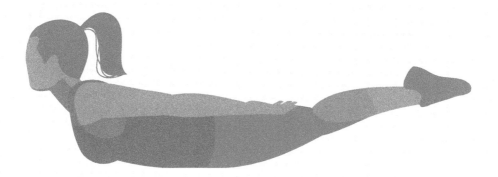

High Knees

1. Start in a standing position.
2. Jog in place, bringing your knees toward your chest (at least as high as your hips), taking deep breaths.

TIP To reduce impact, march in place, bringing your knees up and exhaling with each leg lift.

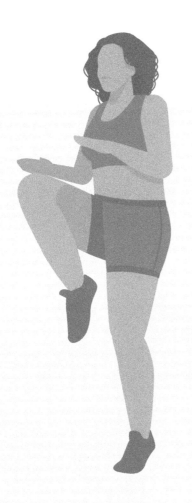
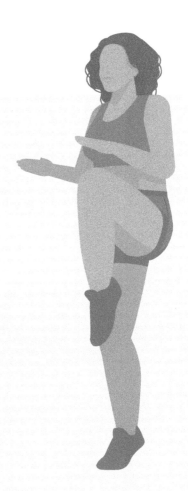

Hip Extension

1. Stand with your knees slightly bent and tap one leg behind you with your toe pointed.

2. Use your glutes to lift your leg off the floor with control and lower it back down.

3. Repeat on the other side.

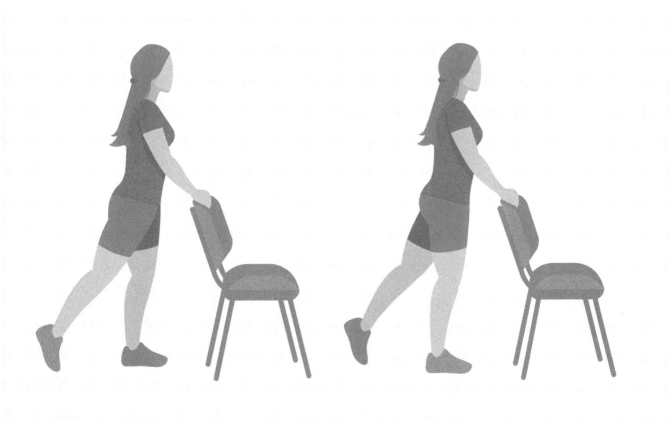

Hip Raise

1. Start on your back with your knees bent and your feet pressing into the floor.

2. Press your hips up toward the ceiling, then lower them down to two inches above the floor.

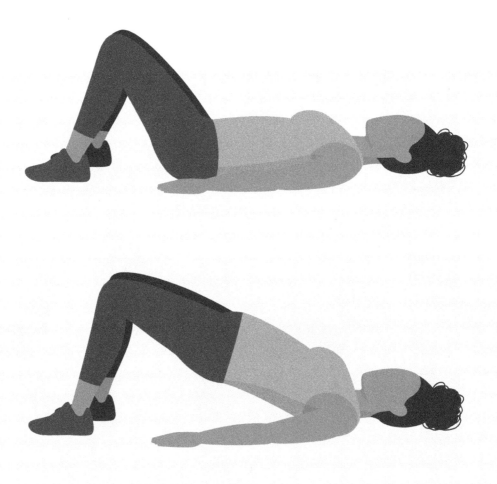

Jump Rope

1. Jump rope like you did as a kid, swinging the rope over your head from behind and jumping over it as it passes under your feet.

2. Do this exercise as quickly as you can, and always remember to land with soft knees.

> **TIP** March or skip in place if you don't have a jump rope.

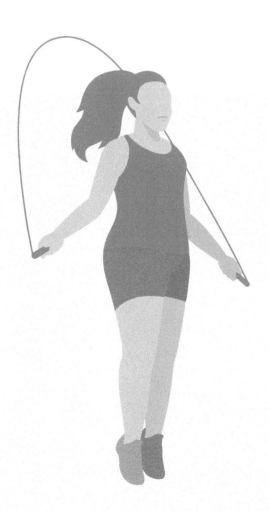

Kettlebell or Dumbbell Swing

1. Stand with your feet hip-width apart and distribute your weight evenly on each foot. Hold the kettlebell between your legs at knee level and start to gently swing it so you can gain momentum.

2. When you're ready, power through your hips, glutes, and core to swing the weight up to shoulder height, then bend your knees, swinging it back to start. Every time the weight goes up, strongly exhale.

TIP Use your glutes and core, *not* your arms, to lift the weight.

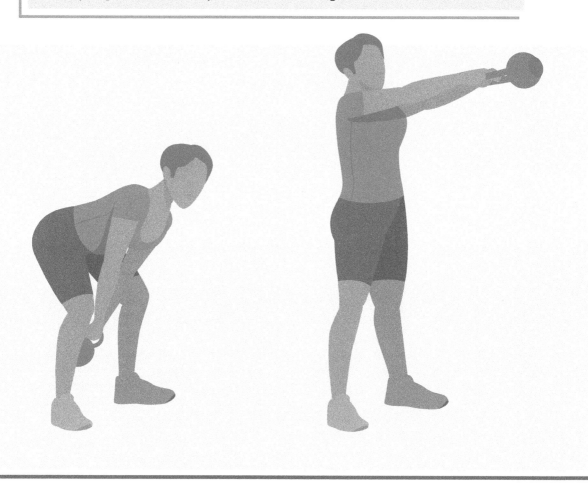

March

1. Start on your back, with your knees bent and feet pressing into the floor. Exhale and lift one leg up, keeping the leg bent at 90 degrees.

2. Lower your leg down with control and repeat on the opposite side. Keep your abs engaged.

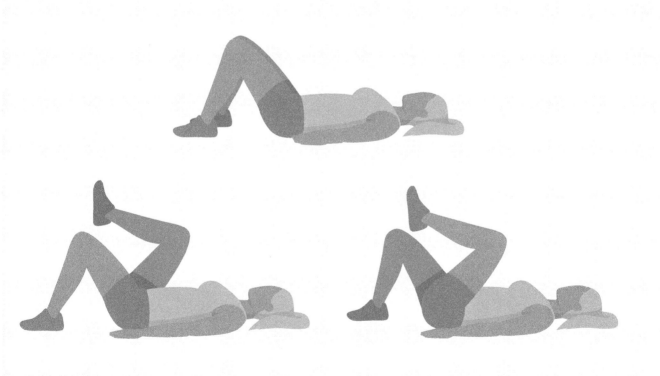

Mountain Climber

1. Get into plank position with your wrists under your shoulders.

2. Bring one knee toward the elbow on the same side. Move back to plank and switch to the opposite side.

> **TIP** For a greater challenge, move as quickly as possible. To reduce core pressure, perform this exercise with your hands on a wall or a sturdy bench.

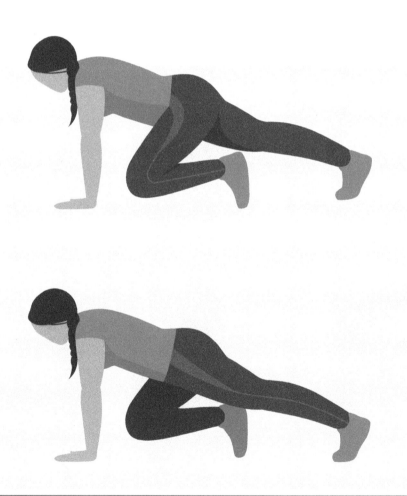

Plank

1. Begin on all fours, stretched out in one long, straight line from your head through your knees or toes (depending on whether you're modifying).

2. If you're on your toes, press back through your heels, and no matter what, keep your hips in line with your spine. Tilt your chin away from your chest so your neck stays long, and take some nice, deep breaths.

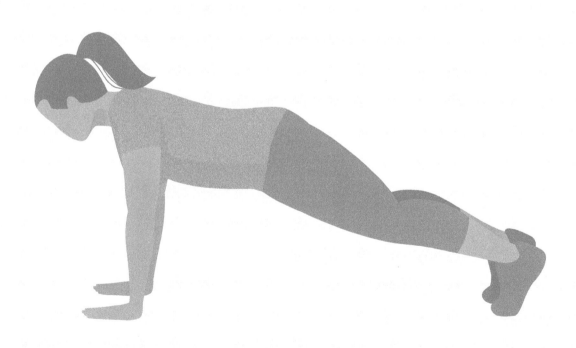

Plank Jack

1. Start in a plank position, with your hands wide and your knuckles pressed into the floor.

2. Walk or jump your feet out, then walk or jump back to plank. You're essentially making a jumping jack movement from the plank position, without your hands leaving the floor.

TIP Try to keep your hips in line with your body and tighten your core.

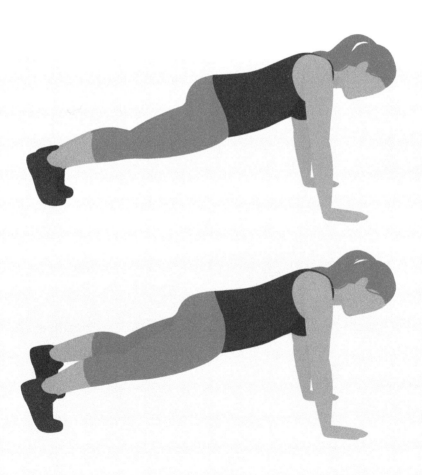

Plank Reach Out and Back

1. Begin on all fours, stretched out in one long, straight line from your head through your knees or toes (depending on whether you're modifying). If you're on your toes, press back through your heels, and no matter what, keep your hips in line with your spine.

2. Tilt your chin away from your chest so your neck stays long, and take some nice, deep breaths.

3. Reach one arm out and inhale. Then as you exhale, press back into downward-facing dog, forming a triangle with your hips at the top point, feet and hands on the ground. On your next inhale, reach toward the opposite ankle.

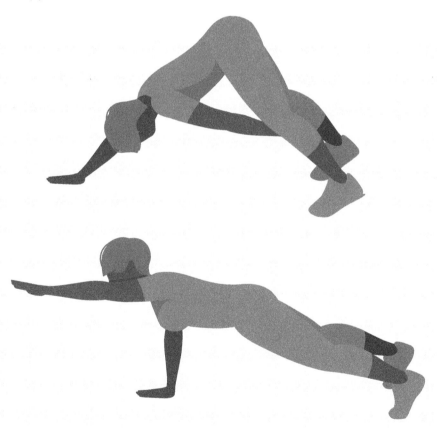

Plié Squat Jump

1. Get into a plié squat position (feet wider than your hips and toes slightly turned out, with your hips down so your thighs are almost parallel to the floor) and put your hands on your hips. Keep your abs engaged and your chest lifted.

2. Powering through your heels, spring up, reaching your arms toward the ceiling. Land with a soft knee. Touch the floor as you squat and repeat.

> **TIP** To reduce impact, eliminate the jump and just reach your arms overhead, coming up onto your toes.

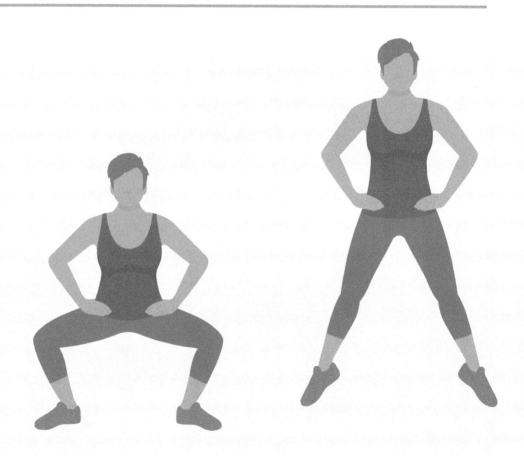

Push-Up

1. Start in a plank position with your arms just to the outside of your shoulders. Bend your elbows toward the floor and stop when they're in line with your torso.

2. Keep your hips down in line with your spine and exhale, squeezing your chest, to rise.

> **TIP** While executing push-ups from your toes is the standard version, you can modify by doing them on your knees or from a standing position, leaning forward with your hands against a wall.

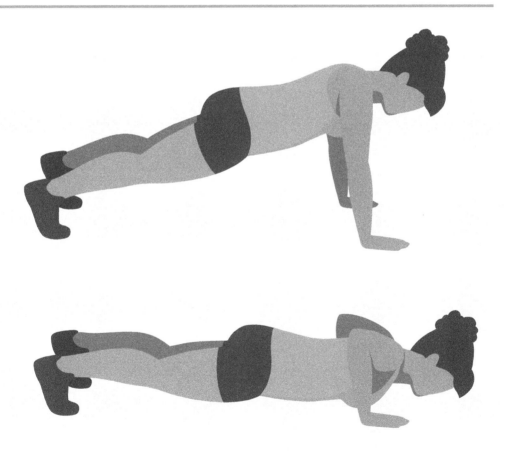

Resistance Band Donkey Kick

1. Loop the resistance band two inches above your knees and come to all fours, hands stacked under your shoulders and knees under your hips. Gaze down toward the floor keeping your neck long.

2. Maintain a bend in the knees and contract your glutes to lift one leg off the floor, pressing your heel toward the ceiling. With control, lower your leg down and exhale as you lift it back up. Keep both hips pointing down toward the floor.

3. Complete your full-range movements, then pulse at the top before switching to the opposite side.

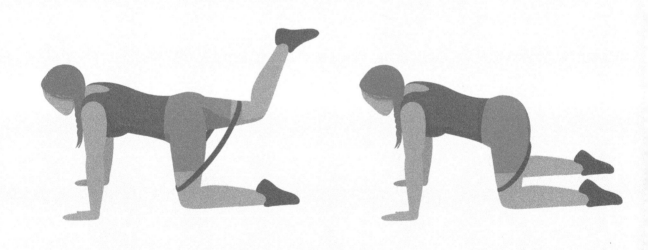

Reverse Lunge

1. Stand hip-width apart and take a big step back with your right foot.

2. Sink down to a lunge position, aiming to create a 90-degree angle with both legs, front knee stacked over your front ankle. Keep your chest lifted and core tight.

3. Place your weight on your front foot as you return to the starting position. Repeat on the opposite side.

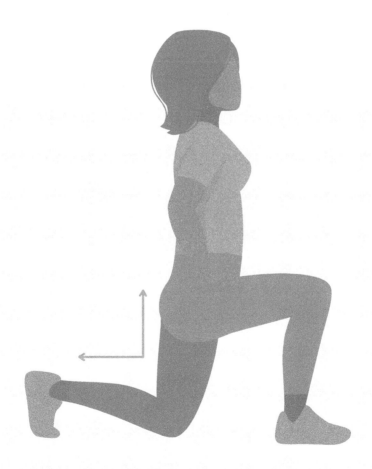

Rotating Squat Jump

1. Stand with your feet shoulder-width apart and sink low into a squat.

2. Jump 180 degrees, and land with a soft knee to squat on the opposite side.

> **TIP** If necessary, start with 90 degrees and build up to the full turn. To reduce impact, walk 180 degrees to squat on the other side.

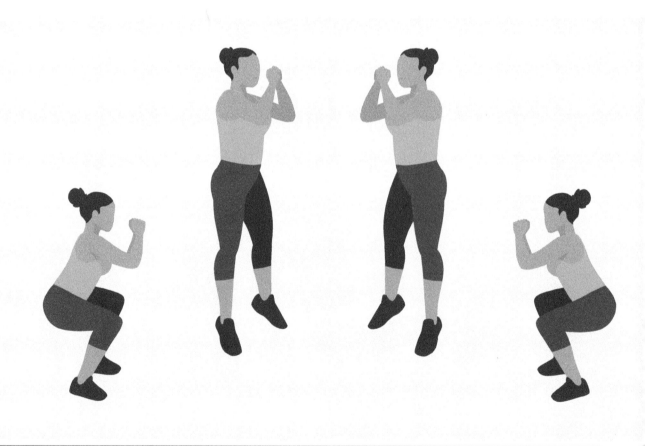

Shoulder Raise

1. Stand with your legs shoulder-width apart holding a pair of dumbbells down by your sides.

2. Keeping a slight bend in your elbows, lift the dumbbells to shoulder height, forming the letter "T," then lower them back down.

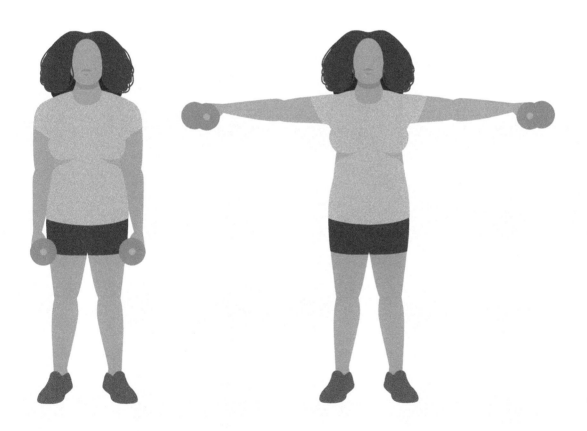

Side Plank

1. Begin in a lying position on your right or left side. Place one hand on the floor directly under your shoulder, or rest on your forearm. You can modify this exercise by placing your bottom knee on the ground.

2. Lift up through your bottom oblique, keeping your entire hand planted on the floor.

3. Stagger your feet for more control, or stack for a balance challenge.

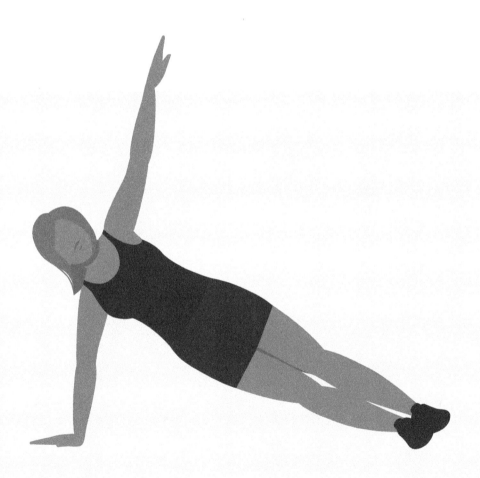

Sit Squat

1. Stand about one foot in front of a sturdy chair or bench, with your back to it. Place your feet just under your hips with your toes slightly angled out.

2. Keep your chest lifted and core tight as you sink back and down into a squat, sitting on the chair or bench for a brief second. Your weight should remain in your heels, and your knees should be directly stacked over your ankles.

3. Exhale and squeeze your glutes to rise.

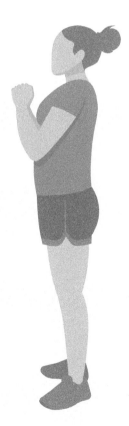
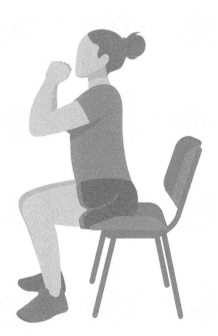

Skater

1. Start with both feet on the ground with one leg forward and your toes angled out 45 degrees.

2. Moving quickly, step your other foot totally back behind the front, so that your foot is behind the opposite shoulder.

3. Sink low into a curtsy lunge (stepping one leg behind the other), rise, and step to repeat on the opposite side.

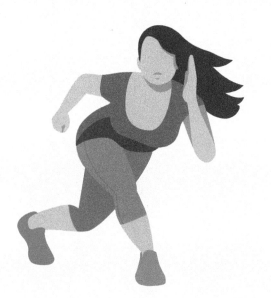
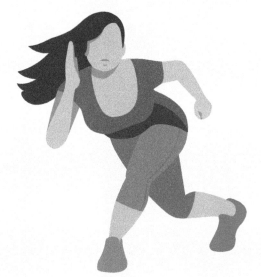

Ski Hop

1. Start with your legs together with a slight bend at the knees.
2. Spring up and jump laterally to the right (about one foot) landing with soft knees.
3. Spring up and jump to the left, landing with slightly bent knees.

TIP To modify, step to the side instead of jumping.

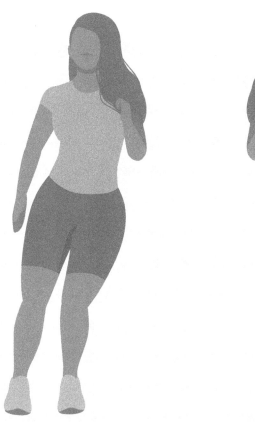
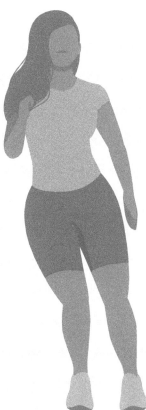

Squat Jump

1. Squat (keep your butt *low* and back). Keep your abs engaged and chest lifted with your feet shoulder-width apart, slightly turned out.

2. Powering through your heels, spring up, arms at your side or reaching toward the ceiling. Land with soft knees, cushioning your landing by letting your legs gently absorb the impact. If possible, bend your legs a minimum of 90 degrees.

> **TIP** To reduce impact, simply do quick bodyweight squats in which you squat with both arms straight out in front of you, keeping your knees directly over your feet as practical.

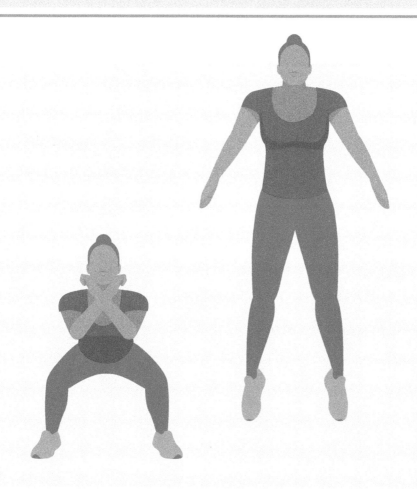

Squat to Overhead Press

1. Stand with your feet a little wider than your hips and your toes turned slightly out.

2. Hold a pair of dumbbells just above your shoulders (for stability, you could bring your hands to your shoulders, elbows pointing forward). Keep your chest lifted and your weight in your heels as you squat, keeping your butt well behind you.

3. Exhale and squeeze your butt to rise, lifting the dumbbells straight up in the air from your shoulders, fully extending your arms before returning the weights to the starting position.

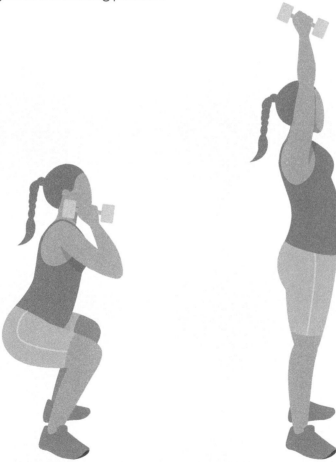

Step-Up

1. Stand about two feet behind a sturdy bench or chair.

2. Place one entire foot (not just the toes) on the bench or chair. Bring the other leg up to meet it.

3. Lower down with control and repeat on the opposite side.

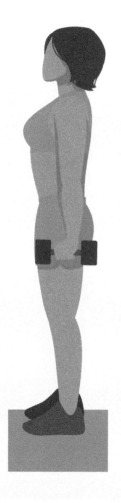
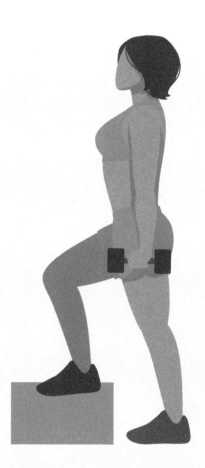

Sumo Squat

1. For this squat variation, start with a *really* wide stance and your toes turned out.

2. As you move into a squat, keep your chest lifted and sink your thighs parallel to the floor. Make sure your knees extend toward, but not past, your toes.

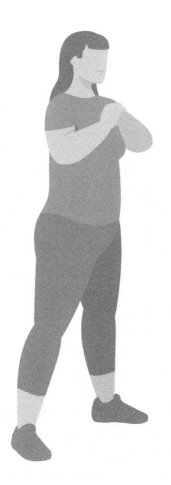
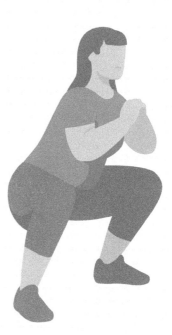

Superwoman

1. Lie down on your stomach. Stretch your body out with your head facing down. Your torso, thighs, and the tops of your feet should be firmly planted on the floor.

2. Extend your arms out in front of you. With the strength of your core and low back, lift your arms and legs off the ground. Keep your gaze down toward the floor.

3. Lower down with control.

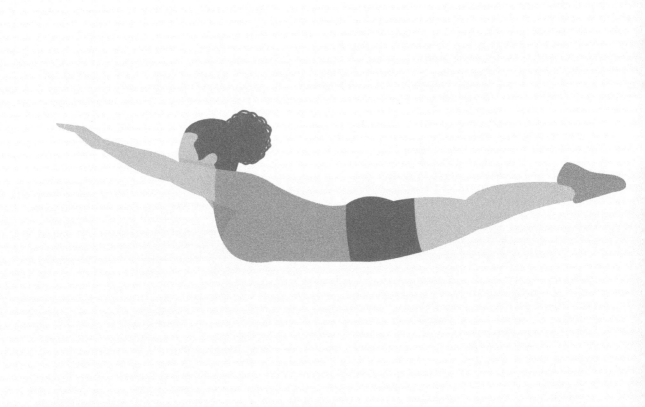

Thruster

1. Squat, planting both hands firmly on the floor.
2. Walk or hop back to a plank position (push-up here is optional), then walk or hop your feet back to your squat.

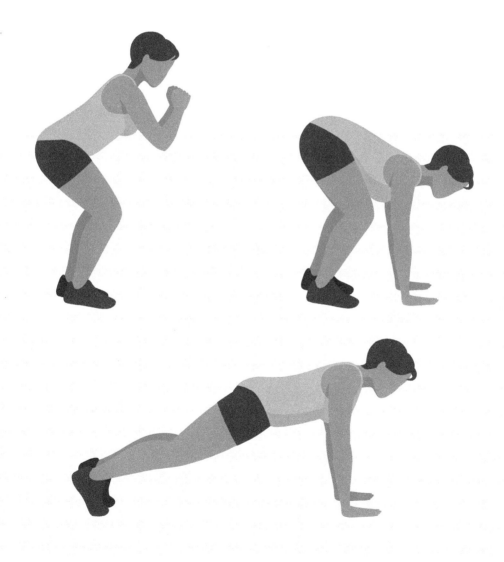

Triceps Dip

1. Place a bench or chair behind you. Sit with your butt directly against the front of the bench. Place your hands behind you, gripping its edge. Either bend your knees with your feet flat on the floor or, for a challenge, straighten your legs in front of you, resting on your heels. (For even more of a challenge, place a flat plate on your legs.)

2. Straighten your arms, but don't lock your elbows. Slowly lower your body toward the floor until your elbows reach a 90-degree angle. Keep your chest lifted and shoulders down.

3. Push back to start.

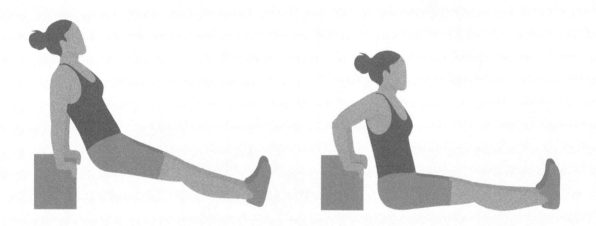

Triceps Extension

1. Place your feet just under your hips with a slight bend at the knees. Hinge slightly forward from your hips, keeping your back flat (shoulders pulled back) and core tight.

2. Bring your elbows in by your sides and use your triceps to straighten your arm toward your back, as if you were trying to pass a baton behind you, before bending and lowering back down.

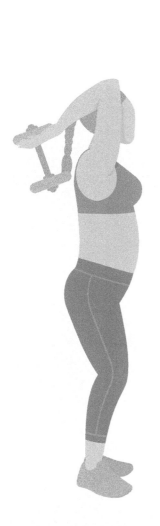
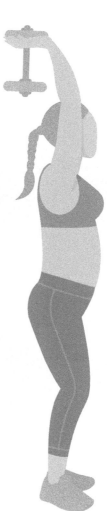

Upright Row

1. Stand with your legs shoulder-width apart and hold a pair of dumbbells down by your sides.
2. Lift your elbows along a horizontal line at shoulder height, arms bent, weights in front of your rib cage.
3. Lower the weights back down.

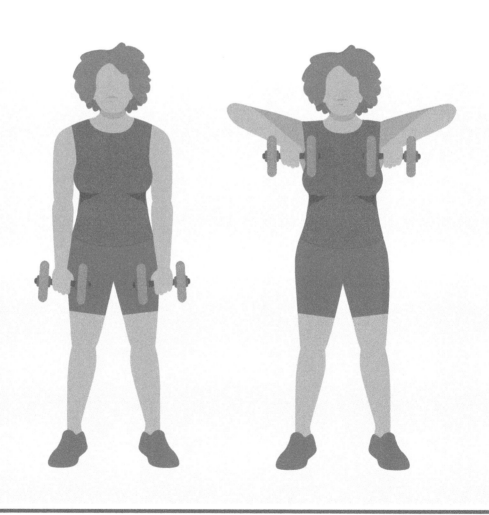

Wall Sit

1. Stand with your back against a wall and slide down until your thighs are parallel to the floor.

2. Make sure your knees don't extend beyond your toes—you may need to walk your feet out a little—and spread your weight evenly throughout your feet.

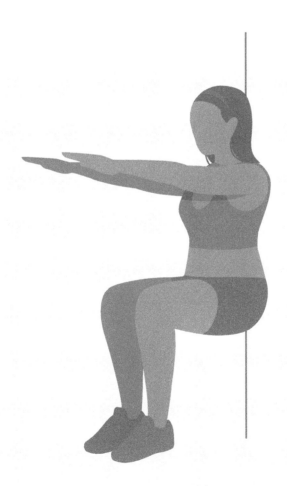

X-Abs

1. Lie on your back with your arms and legs out in an "X" shape.

2. Lift one arm and the opposite leg up, reaching your arm toward your toes. Lower them back down to the floor and repeat on the other side.

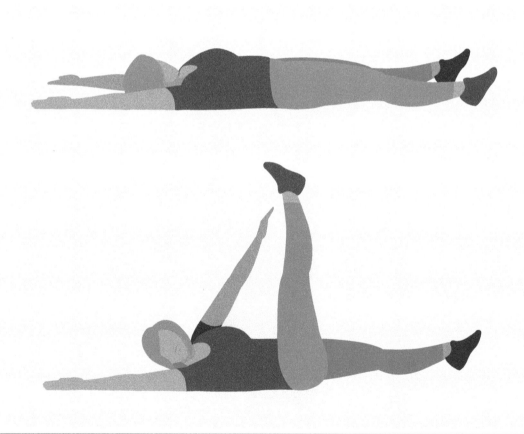

X-Jump

1. From a standing position, jump your legs out as if you were doing a jumping jack, as you reach one hand to the ground between your feet.

2. Stand back up as you jump your legs closed, then jump your legs out and touch the ground with your other hand.

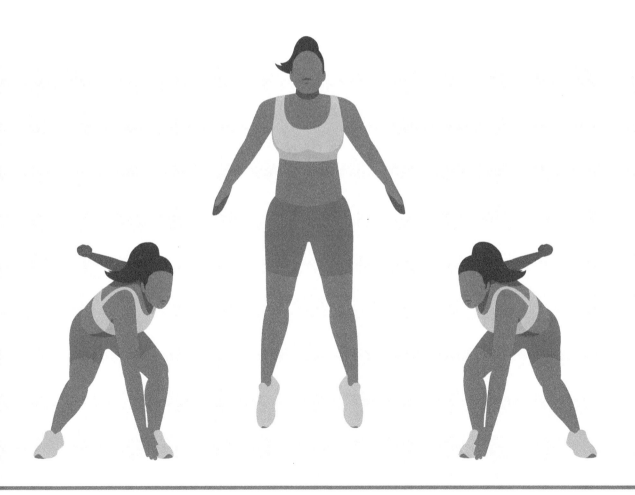

Cool Downs

The cool-down portion of a workout allows the body to return to homeostasis. Heart rate, breathing rate, and tissue temperature all decrease, and our bodies consume excess oxygen. A cool-down period can also help keep your blood pressure from dropping too rapidly and blood pooling in the lower body, which can lead to dizziness and fainting. After your workout, take time to slow down your pace and intensity while taking deep breaths. One of the best cool-down methods is simply to walk for five minutes at a moderate pace, slowing down the walking speed each minute. Afterward, do some static stretches modeled after the workout you just completed—do some upper body stretches following a challenging arm workout, for instance.

Note: All static stretches should be held for 15 to 25 seconds, and repeated on the opposite limb/side (if applicable). You should feel a constant pressure that's never painful when you're stretching. Don't incorporate a pulsing or repetitive movement to get deeper into the stretch.

UPPER BODY

- **Chest stretch:** From a standing position, drape your arms behind your back and interlace your fingers with your knuckles toward the floor. Slowly bend at the waist while rotating your straightened arms away from your body until you feel a gentle stretch at your chest.

- **Low back release:** Hold on to a sturdy countertop. Walk your feet back until your back is parallel to the floor and your arms are straight. Take a deep breath and pull away from the countertop, feeling a stretch through your back and shoulders.

- **Shoulder stretch:** From a standing position, fully extend your arm and bring it across your chest parallel to the ground. Using your other arm, cradle the original arm just behind your elbow on the triceps side in order to support the arm and provide a slight pressure for a stretch you should feel in your shoulder.

- **Triceps stretch:** From a standing position, extend both arms directly above your head perpendicular to the ground. From that position, rotate one forearm down and behind your head, pointing as far toward the ground as feels comfortable. Place the hand of the other arm on top of your stretching arm's elbow and gently pull.

LOWER BODY

- **Calf stretch:** There are several variations of this stretch, but here's a good version for beginners. Stand with your feet shoulder-width apart with a slight bend in the knees. Slide one foot back until it's approximately a foot or so behind the heel of the other foot. Straighten your back foot and lean slightly forward so you feel a comfortable tension in your calf. You can adjust your forward foot, moving it even more forward, to deepen the stretch.

- **Glutes/piriformis stretch:** From a seated position with both legs extended in front of you, cross your right ankle above your left knee and flex from your foot. Bend your left leg, sliding your left foot toward your body until you feel a stretch in your glutes. Hold it here and breathe.

- **Hamstring stretch:** From a standing position with your feet and knees together, bend at the hip and attempt to touch your toes with extended fingers. A slight bend in the knees is fine. If you can't touch your toes, simply reach as far as you can without causing pain. You can also do this stretch from a seated position.

- **Quadriceps stretch:** Get into a standing position from which you can comfortably balance on one foot. Rotate one leg at the knee to a position directly behind that leg, and grab your foot with the hand on that same side. Attempt to keep your body upright with your chest high, feeling a slight pressure in your hamstring in front of your leg. If you find it difficult to keep your balance, try focusing on a non-moving object on the ground.

FULL BODY

- **Kneeling reach:** From a kneeling position, place your right foot forward and flat on the floor, making sure your right knee is stacked over your right ankle. Gently press your hips forward to feel a nice stretch in your hip flexors, and reach your arms overhead. Drop your shoulders and breathe. Repeat on the opposite side.

- **Spinal twist:** From a seated and cross-legged position, place your left hand on your right knee. Gently twist your torso toward the right, keeping a tall posture and both shoulders pressing down. Repeat on the opposite side.

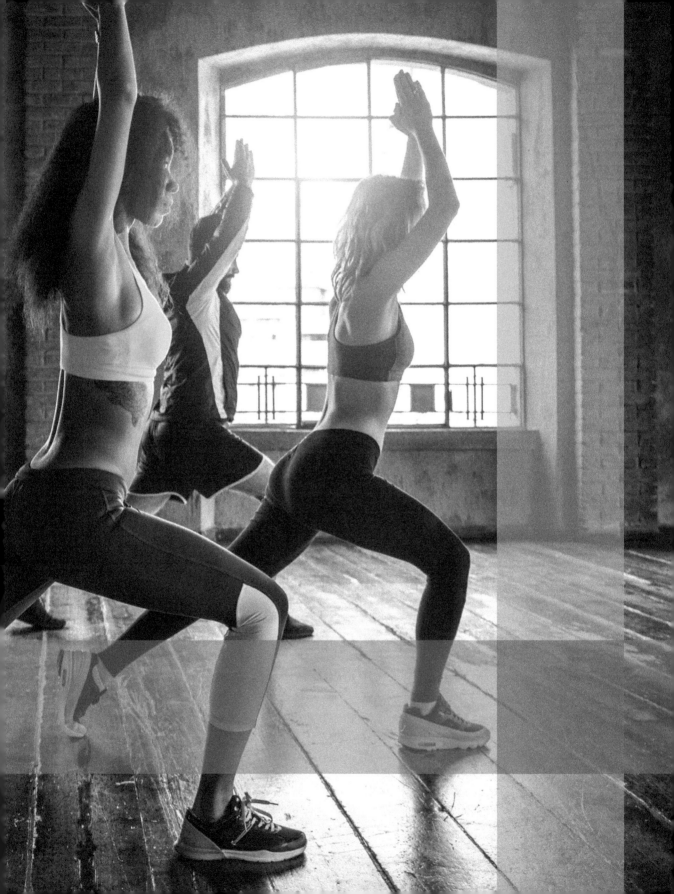

CHAPTER THREE

The Workouts

It's time to get started with effective workouts you can complete in 15 minutes using minimal equipment. These workouts are designed to help you maximize your fitness results in a place of your choosing. They are divided into the following categories:

- Core, arms, and abs

- Legs and glutes

- Full body

These workouts include tips for modifications, numbered steps, and illustrations to help ensure proper form. They progress in difficulty, so follow each section's workouts in sequence. It's absolutely okay—in fact it's recommended—to repeat workouts, not least because it's a great way to gauge your progress and see how much stronger you get over time.

Before you proceed with this exercise regimen, remember that it's not a good idea to do HIIT workouts every day. Your heart is a muscle that needs adequate time to repair and recover. Alternating the intensity levels of your workouts throughout the week—scheduling an easier workout the day after a challenging one—helps your whole body recover. A good rule of thumb: If you did it yesterday, don't do it again today.

I've included some purely strength-based workouts to alternate with HIIT exercises and cardio-focused workouts. If you have a challenging HIIT day, go for a walk or easy run the following day or try a strength workout. The next day, you'll be ready for more HIIT. Generally speaking, I don't recommend doing cardio-driven HIIT workouts more than three times a week on non-consecutive days.

Here are some examples of weekly schedules based on how many days you have available to exercise:

- Two days per week: two full-body workouts on non-consecutive days; or one day of core, arms, and abs and one day of legs and glutes workout

- Three days per week: three full-body workouts on non-consecutive days; or one day of core, arms, and abs, one day of legs and glutes, and one full-body workout

- Four days per week: two days of core, arms, and abs and two days of legs and glutes; or one day of core, arms, and abs, one day of legs and glutes, and two full-body workouts on non-consecutive days

- Five days per week: one day of easy cardio of choice, two days of core, arms, and abs, and two days of legs and glutes; or one day of core, arms, and abs, one day of legs and glutes, two full-body workouts on non-consecutive days, and one day of easy cardio of choice

No matter your workout schedule, always allow at least one to two days per week of full rest. On these days, go for a walk around the neighborhood or enjoy some restorative self-care: Meditate, have a bubble bath, take a nap, or do whatever feels restorative to you. This practice allows your body to recover for the following week.

Core, Arms, and Abs

It's a common misconception to think of the core solely as your abdominal muscles. Your entire torso area is your core.

Core strength is incredibly important because we use our core for many everyday activities. The core helps keep the torso strong; supports the back as we hinge forward, arch backward, or twist; promotes balance, which prevents falls as we age; and supports the body in all planes of movement. Essentially, all exercises (and virtually all movements throughout the day) are based on the foundation of a well-developed core.

A strong core can also help prevent back pain, promote good posture and alignment, and assist supporting structures (like the glutes and pelvic floor that are, indeed, parts of the core). In this section, I've also included exercises for arms (for lifting and holding heavy items) and some isolated abdominals exercises.

By doing smart core training, you'll be able to create visible tone and muscular development as well as develop a good foundation.

Arm Burner

This workout combines some great HIIT exercises with arm work for a sweaty and fun workout.

 # OF CIRCUITS X DURATION 3 rounds, 1 minute per exercise

TOTAL WORKOUT TIME 15 minutes

TOTAL TIME 25 minutes, including warm-up, workout, and cool down

WARM-UP 5 minutes with a quick functional circuit or moderate cardio of choice

RECOVERY 30 seconds, if needed

COOL DOWN 5 minutes (page 56)

COMMON MISTAKES AND HOW TO AVOID THEM Don't move too quickly through the exercises. Take your time and breathe during the strength components. It will feel like a nice recovery so you're ready to go for the next HIIT round.

CHANGE IT UP To modify the push-ups, place your hands on a wall or a countertop. If you don't have a jump rope, feel free to jog in place or march with high knees. For an extra challenge, hold heavier weights for the biceps curls.

HIIT Circuit (3 rounds, 1 minute per exercise)

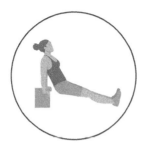

1. TRICEPS DIP, PAGE 50

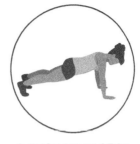

2. PUSH-UP, PAGE 35

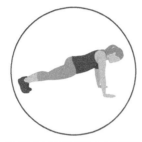

3. PLANK JACK, PAGE 32

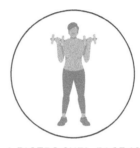

4. BICEPS CURL, PAGE 19

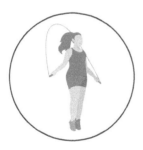

**5. JUMP ROPE, PAGE 27,
(OR SKIP IN PLACE)**

Core on Fire

This workout combines HIIT intervals with abdominal work to strengthen your core while still working up a great sweat.

 # OF CIRCUITS X DURATION 3 rounds, 1 minute per exercise

TOTAL WORKOUT TIME 15 minutes

TOTAL TIME 25 minutes, including warm-up, workout, and cool down

WARM-UP 5 minutes with a quick functional circuit or moderate cardio of choice

RECOVERY 30 seconds, if needed

COOL DOWN 5 minutes (page 56)

COMMON MISTAKES AND HOW TO AVOID THEM Start with the low-impact version of each exercise before progressing to higher-impact.

HIIT Circuit (3 rounds, 1 minute per exercise)

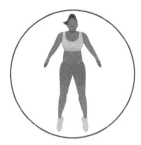

1. X-JUMP, PAGE 55

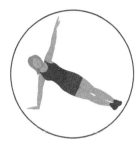

2. SIDE PLANK, PAGE 40, (30 SECONDS EACH SIDE)

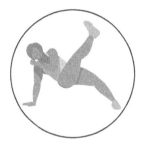

3. BREAKDANCER, PAGE 20

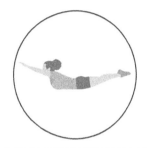

4. SUPERWOMAN, PAGE 48

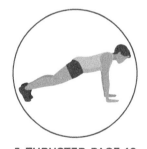

5. THRUSTER, PAGE 49

Arm AMRAP

This workout is meant to be completed AMRAP style, completing "as many rounds as possible" within 15 minutes. See if you can increase the number each time.

 # OF CIRCUITS X DURATION Do as many rounds as possible in 15 minutes. Set a timer and work through each round.

TOTAL WORKOUT TIME 15 minutes

TOTAL TIME 25 minutes, including warm-up, workout, and cool down

WARM-UP 5 minutes with a quick functional circuit or moderate cardio of choice

RECOVERY Minimize rest during the 15-minute time block, but take a breather when needed.

COOL DOWN 5 minutes (page 56)

COMMON MISTAKES AND HOW TO AVOID THEM Don't sacrifice form for speed. Take the time to breathe and correctly set up each movement.

REMEMBER Move quickly and efficiently. If you need to modify the exercise to keep going, please do so.

CHANGE IT UP There are several ways to modify this workout. You can separate the squat and press (10 squats followed by 10 overhead presses) or use lighter weights to minimize the impact; for the burpee, "walk" your feet to plank position and back to your hands instead of jumping. For an advanced version of this circuit, hold heavier weights for the squat to overhead press and shoulder raise. You could also add a tuck jump (raising your knees to your chest as you spring up) at the top of the burpee.

ARMRAP Circuit (15 minutes, AMRAP)

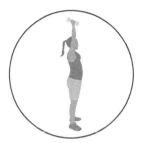

1. SQUAT TO OVERHEAD PRESS, PAGE 45, X 10 REPS

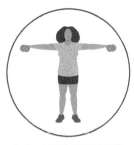

2. SHOULDER RAISE, PAGE 39, X 10 REPS

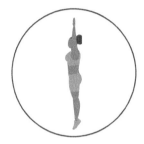

3. BURPEE, PAGE 21, X 5 REPS

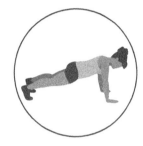

4. PUSH-UP, PAGE 35, X 10 REPS

Arm and HIIT Blitz

This workout includes rest intervals. You're working as hard as you can for 45 seconds and resting for 15 seconds before moving on to the next move. Try to really challenge yourself during the work intervals because you have a built-in rest.

 # OF CIRCUITS X DURATION 3 rounds, 1 minute per exercise (45 seconds of work and 15 seconds of rest)

TOTAL WORKOUT TIME 15 minutes

TOTAL TIME 25 minutes, including warm-up, workout, and cool down

WARM-UP 5 minutes with a quick functional circuit or moderate cardio of choice

RECOVERY Because you're working for 45 seconds and resting for 15 seconds before moving on to the next exercise, recovery is built in.

COOL DOWN 5 minutes (page 56)

COMMON MISTAKES AND HOW TO AVOID THEM For the swings, remember the movement is coming from your glutes and core with a strong exhale, not from arm strength. You may need a heavier weight than you think!

REMEMBER Keep your core engaged and exhale on the work part of each movement.

CHANGE IT UP To reduce impact, eliminate the jump in the rotating squat jumps. Instead, walk to one side, squat, and walk to the other side, squat. You can also bend your knees or do marches for the X-abs.

HIIT Circuit (3 rounds, 1 minute per exercise)

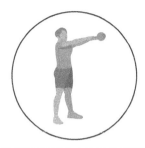

1. KETTLEBELL OR DUMBBELL SWING, PAGE 28

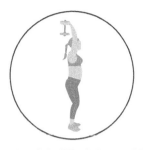

2. TRICEPS EXTENSION, PAGE 51

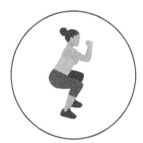

3. ROTATING SQUAT JUMP, PAGE 38

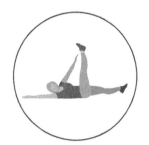

4. X-ABS, PAGE 54

Core Crusher

This workout is a great way to challenge your core while also working up a great sweat in the HIIT intervals, all in just 15 minutes.

 # OF CIRCUITS X DURATION 3 rounds, 1 minute per exercise

TOTAL WORKOUT TIME 15 minutes

TOTAL TIME 25 minutes, including warm-up, workout, and cool down

WARM-UP 5 minutes with a quick functional circuit or moderate cardio of choice

RECOVERY 30 seconds to 1 minute before moving on to the next round

COOL DOWN 5 minutes (page 56)

COMMON MISTAKES AND HOW TO AVOID THEM Because we're focusing on pure core for this workout, take the time to ensure your core is engaged and you're breathing.

CHANGE IT UP To reduce impact, replace the ski hops with bodyweight squats (squats with both arms straight out in front of you, keeping your knees directly over your feet as much as you can). Instead of the high knees, march in place, and rather than plank jacks, place your hands on a wall or a countertop and "walk" your feet out instead of jumping. For more intensity, move more quickly and explosively, or place a weight on your lower abdomen for the hip raises.

Strength and HIIT Circuit (3 rounds, 1 minute per exercise)

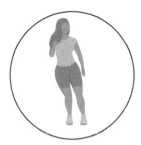

1. SKI HOP, PAGE 43

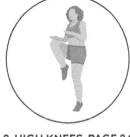

2. HIGH KNEES, PAGE 24

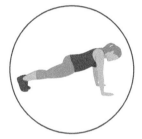

3. PLANK JACK, PAGE 32

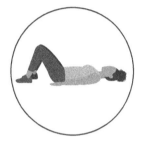

4. HIP RAISE, PAGE 26

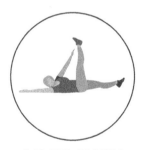

5. X-ABS , PAGE 54

Sun's Out, Guns Out

This workout was designed to challenge your upper body with burner rounds. You'll work the same muscle group twice in a row before moving on to the next muscle group. Fully fatiguing each group in this way improves long-term strength and endurance.

 # OF CIRCUITS X DURATION This workout is meant to be completed AMRAP style, as many rounds as possible in 15 minutes. Set a timer and work through each round. Because this workout is more strength-based, do it the day before or after a more challenging HIIT workout.

TOTAL WORKOUT TIME 15 minutes

TOTAL TIME 25 minutes, including warm-up, workout, and cool down

WARM-UP 5 minutes with a quick functional circuit or moderate cardio of choice

RECOVERY 30 seconds, if needed, before moving on to the next round

COOL DOWN 5 minutes (page 56)

COMMON MISTAKES AND HOW TO AVOID THEM Use weights that will challenge you while allowing proper form. The first time you do this workout, choose weights that seem a little too light. Better to start off too light and build from there than use weights so heavy they're unsafe.

CHANGE IT UP To modify the push-ups, do them on your knees or with your hands on a wall or a countertop. For more of a challenge, hold heavier weights.

Strength Circuit (15 minutes, AMRAP)

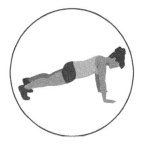

1. PUSH-UP, PAGE 35, X 12 REPS

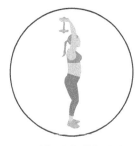

2. TRICEPS EXTENSION, PAGE 51, X 12 REPS

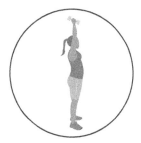

3. SQUAT TO OVERHEAD PRESS, PAGE 45, X 12 REPS

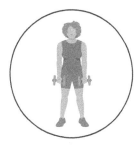

4. UPRIGHT ROW, PAGE 52, X 12 REPS

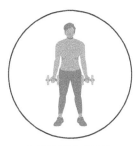

5. BICEPS CURL, PAGE 19, X 12 REPS

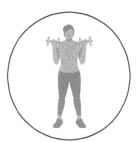

6. BICEPS CURL PULSE, PAGE 19, X 20 REPS

Arm and Abs Shredder

This workout consists of strength work with a round of squat jumps at the end of each set to elevate the heart rate. When your heart rate is elevated from a little blast of cardio, you'll burn more calories during the strength rounds.

 # OF CIRCUITS X DURATION This workout is meant to be completed AMRAP style, as many rounds as possible in 15 minutes. Set a timer and work through each round. Because this workout is strength-based, do it the day before or after a more challenging HIIT workout.

TOTAL WORKOUT TIME 15 minutes

TOTAL TIME 25 minutes, including warm-up, workout, and cool down

WARM-UP 5 minutes with a quick functional circuit or moderate cardio of choice

RECOVERY 30 seconds, if needed, before moving on to the next round

COOL DOWN 5 minutes (page 56)

COMMON MISTAKES AND HOW TO AVOID THEM Don't raise the weights above shoulder height or lock your elbows. Instead, stop the weights at shoulder height and keep a slight bend at the elbows. Lower the weights down in a controlled way, instead of letting the weights drop your arms down.

CHANGE IT UP To modify the push-ups, do them on your knees or with your hands on a wall or a countertop. For more of a challenge, hold heavier weights.

Strength Circuit (15 minutes, AMRAP)

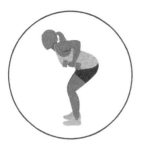

**1. BENT-OVER ROW,
PAGE 18, X 15 REPS**

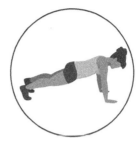

2. PUSH-UP, PAGE 35, X 15 REPS

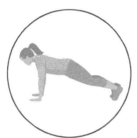

**3. PLANK, PAGE 31,
X 30 SECONDS**

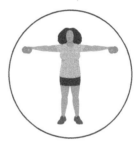

**4. SHOULDER RAISE,
PAGE 39, X 15 REPS**

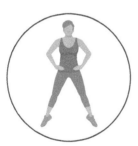

**5. PLIÉ SQUAT JUMP,
PAGE 34, X 20 REPS**

Can't Stop, Won't Stop Arms and Abs

This workout focuses on endurance, using lighter weights and more reps, and changes the traditional muscle-building (hypertrophy-based) strength work. Hypertrophy workouts use 10 to 12 reps; endurance exercises use lighter weights and 12 to 25 reps. Endurance exercises prepare your muscles to work for the long haul, whether for racing or carrying grocery bags.

 # OF CIRCUITS X DURATION This workout is meant to be completed AMRAP style, as many rounds as possible in 15 minutes. Set a timer and work through each round. Because this workout is more strength-based, do it the day before or after a more challenging HIIT workout.

TOTAL WORKOUT TIME 15 minutes

TOTAL TIME 25 minutes, including warm-up, workout, and cool down

WARM-UP 5 minutes with a quick functional circuit or moderate cardio of choice

RECOVERY 30 seconds, if needed, before moving on to the next round

COOL DOWN 5 minutes (page 56)

COMMON MISTAKES AND HOW TO AVOID THEM Don't hyperextend your back during the Superwoman exercise. Focus on length instead of height.

CHANGE IT UP Start on all fours (hands under your shoulders and knees underneath your hips), and reach out with your right arm while lifting your left leg off the floor and pressing it back. With control, switch sides. For more of a challenge, hold heavier weights.

Strength Circuit (15 minutes, AMRAP)

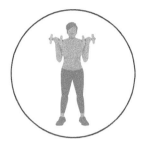

1. BICEPS CURL, PAGE 19, X 20 REPS

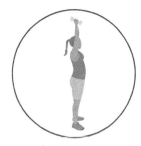

2. SQUAT TO OVERHEAD PRESS, PAGE 45, X 20 REPS

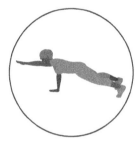

3. PLANK REACH OUT AND BACK, PAGE 33, X 20 REPS TOTAL

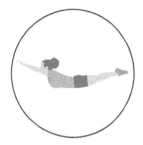

4. SUPERWOMAN, PAGE 48, X 20 REPS

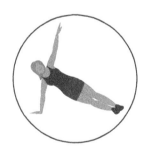

5. SIDE PLANK, PAGE 40, X 30 SECONDS EACH SIDE

Arm and HIIT Power Blast

This workout focuses on endurance, using lighter weights and more reps than hypertrophy-based strength work. Endurance exercises prepare your muscles to work for the long haul, whether for running races or carrying grocery bags.

 # OF CIRCUITS X DURATION This workout is meant to be completed AMRAP style, as many rounds as possible in 15 minutes. Set a timer and work through each round.

TOTAL WORKOUT TIME 15 minutes

TOTAL TIME 25 minutes, including warm-up, workout, and cool down

WARM-UP 5 minutes with a quick functional circuit or moderate cardio of choice

RECOVERY 30 seconds to 1 minute before moving on to the next round

COOL DOWN 5 minutes (page 56)

COMMON MISTAKES AND HOW TO AVOID THEM Keep your back flat and neck long during the triceps extensions.

CHANGE IT UP If you don't have a jump rope, jog or do high knees in place. To modify the burpee, place your hands on a wall. You can also walk your feet back to plank, then back to your hands instead of jumping. For more of a challenge, add a tuck jump (raising your knees to your chest as you spring up) at the top of your burpee.

Strength and HIIT Circuit (15 minutes, AMRAP)

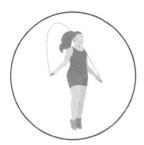

**1. JUMP ROPE, PAGE 27,
X 100 REPS**

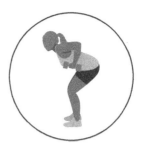

**2. BENT-OVER ROW,
PAGE 18, X 12 REPS**

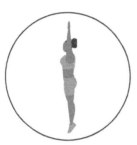

**3. BURPEE, PAGE 21,
X 10 REPS**

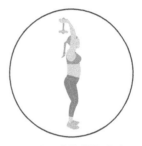

**4. TRICEPS EXTENSION,
PAGE 51, X 12 REPS**

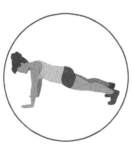

**5. PUSH-UP, PAGE 35,
(MAX 1 MINUTE)**

Give Planks Workout

For visible upper body results, try this circuit. At the end of each exercise, you'll "give planks" with a one-minute plank. Plank any way you'd like and take mini breaks, if needed, during the minute.

 # OF CIRCUITS X DURATION 3 rounds, 1 minute per exercise

TOTAL WORKOUT TIME 12 minutes

TOTAL TIME 22 minutes includes warm-up and cool down

WARM-UP 5 minutes with a quick functional circuit or moderate cardio of choice

RECOVERY 30 seconds, if needed, before moving on to the next round

COOL DOWN 5 minutes (page 56)

COMMON MISTAKES AND HOW TO AVOID THEM In plank position, keep your spine long, neck straight (not kinked), and core pulled in. Breathe.

REMEMBER Each exercise should be done for an entire minute. Take your time to execute each move with proper form.

CHANGE IT UP Modify your plank and push-up by performing them on your knees, if needed. For more of a challenge, hold heavier weights for the squat to overhead press.

Strength and HIIT Circuit (3 rounds, 1 minute per exercise)

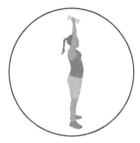

1. SQUAT TO OVERHEAD PRESS, PAGE 45

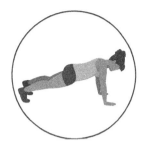

2. PUSH-UP, PAGE 35

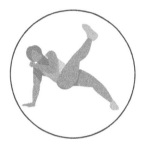

3. BREAKDANCER, PAGE 20

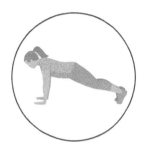

4. PLANK, PAGE 31

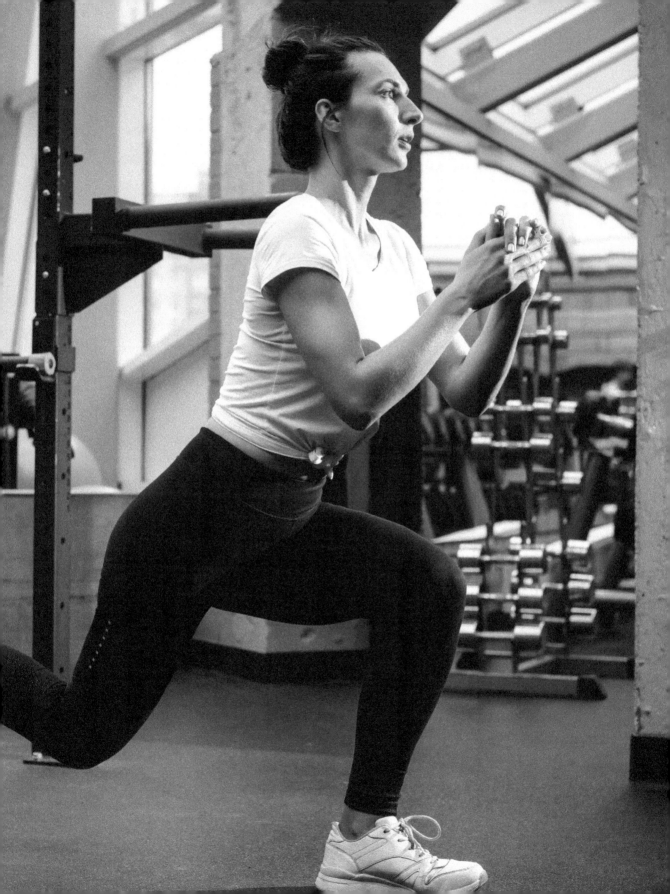

Legs and Glutes

This exercise section is my favorite of the entire book. Legs and glutes are so important for strength training, especially because many of us are weak in these areas. It's easy to think that these larger muscle groups are very strong, yet, in reality, they're underutilized. Most of us spend much of our time in a seated position, which leads to very tight hip flexors and relaxed, weak glute muscles. Strong glutes can help support our core and pelvic floor as well as the lower back, reducing back pain.

In general, the workouts and exercises that help strengthen legs and glutes don't need to be different for women and men—we all need strong bums, after all. But because women can have less muscle mass overall than men, they, especially, need to maintain strength in the legs and glutes over time.

Lunch Break Leg Workout

This is a quick and fun workout to challenge and strengthen your lower body. All you need is a pair of dumbbells.

 # OF CIRCUITS X DURATION 3 rounds, 1 minute per exercise

TOTAL WORKOUT TIME 12 minutes

TOTAL TIME 22 minutes including warm-up, workout, and cool down

WARM-UP 5 minutes with a quick functional circuit or moderate cardio of choice

RECOVERY 30 seconds, if needed, before moving on to the next round

COOL DOWN 5 minutes (page 56)

COMMON MISTAKES AND HOW TO AVOID THEM For your lunges, keep your front knee stacked directly over your front ankle. Think about sinking straight down instead of forward.

CHANGE IT UP Modify the ski hop by doing bodyweight squats (page 44). To eliminate impact from the plié squat jump, just do plié squats. For more of a challenge, hold dumbbells for the step-ups and alternating lunges.

Strength and HIIT Circuit (3 rounds, 1 minute per exercise)

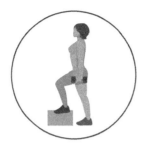

**1. STEP-UP, PAGE 46,
(30 SECONDS EACH SIDE)**

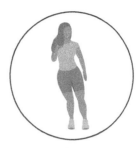

2. SKI HOP, PAGE 43

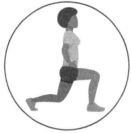

**3. ALTERNATING LUNGE, PAGE 17,
(30 SECONDS EACH SIDE)**

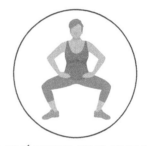

4. PLIÉ SQUAT JUMP, PAGE 34

Leg Strength for Days

This workout does not have explosive intervals, so feel free to do it the day before or after a more challenging HIIT workout, like one that's pure cardio or works the upper body. Move through the exercises with control and good breath work.

 # OF CIRCUITS X DURATION This workout is meant to be completed AMRAP style, as many rounds as possible in 15 minutes. Set a timer and work through each round.

TOTAL WORKOUT TIME 15 minutes

TOTAL TIME 25 minutes, including warm-up, workout, and cool down

WARM-UP 5 minutes with a quick functional circuit or moderate cardio of choice

RECOVERY 30 seconds to 1 minute, if needed, before moving on to the next round

COOL DOWN 5 minutes (page 56)

COMMON MISTAKES AND HOW TO AVOID THEM When you use a resistance band, don't place it directly over your knee. Go for two inches above (my preference) or below the knee.

CHANGE IT UP To decrease the intensity, hold lighter weights or perform the exercises without the resistance band and dumbbells entirely. To increase the intensity of the sit squat, hold a weight or two dumbbells at your chest or use a stronger resistance band. For the hip raise, you can hold a weight on your lower abdomen.

Strength Workout (15 minutes, AMRAP)

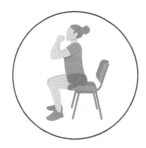

1. SIT SQUAT, PAGE 41, X 15 REPS

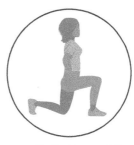

2. REVERSE LUNGE, PAGE 37, X 10 REPS

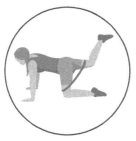

3. RESISTANCE BAND DONKEY KICK, PAGE 36, X 15 REPS

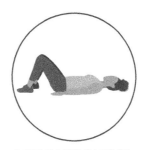

4. HIP RAISE, PAGE 26, X 15 REPS

Perfect Peach HIIT

This workout combines strength training moves with explosive HIIT intervals to increase your heart rate and work up an awesome sweat. All you need is your own body weight.

 # OF CIRCUITS X DURATION 3 rounds, 1 minute of exercise (45 seconds of work, 15 seconds of rest)

TOTAL WORKOUT TIME 15 minutes

TOTAL TIME 25 minutes, including warm-up, workout, and cool down

WARM-UP 5 minutes with a quick functional circuit or moderate cardio of choice

RECOVERY 30 seconds, if needed, before moving on to the next round

COOL DOWN 5 minutes (page 56)

COMMON MISTAKES AND HOW TO AVOID THEM When squatting, people commonly shoot their knees forward. Think about sitting back and down, as if there were a chair behind you.

CHANGE IT UP For the close squats and lunges, opt for dumbbells to make it more challenging. To modify the HIIT intervals, try a slow curtsy lunge (page 42) instead of the skater, ditch the jumps in thruster and squat jumps, walk your feet back to the plank position then to your hands for the thruster, and perform bodyweight squats (page 44) instead of squat jumps.

Strength and HIIT Workout (3 rounds, 1 minute of exercise)

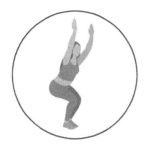

1. CLOSE SQUAT, PAGE 22

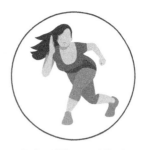

2. SKATER, PAGE 42

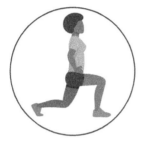

3. LUNGE TO PAUSE, PAGE 17

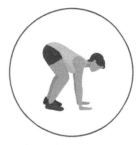

4. THRUSTER, PAGE 49

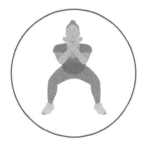

5. SQUAT JUMP, PAGE 44

Booty Burning HIIT

This workout is all sweaty cardio-based movements! It's a great way to get in a short and effective cardio workout.

 # OF CIRCUITS X DURATION 3 rounds, 1 minute of exercise (45 seconds of work, 15 seconds of rest)

TOTAL WORKOUT TIME 15 minutes

TOTAL TIME 25 minutes, including warm-up, workout, and cool down

WARM-UP 5 minutes with a quick functional circuit or moderate cardio of choice

RECOVERY 30 seconds, if needed, before moving on to the next round

COOL DOWN 5 minutes (page 56)

COMMON MISTAKES AND HOW TO AVOID THEM It's easy to start out too fast and burn out with this one. Pace yourself at the beginning of each round so you can keep moving the entire time.

REMEMBER Land with soft knees any time you jump.

CHANGE IT UP To reduce impact, eliminate the jumps. Walk your feet out for the jumping jack portion of the X-jumps and plank jacks. Walk your feet back to plank and back to your hands for the burpees, or perform these with your hands on a wall.

Strength and HIIT Workout (3 rounds, 1 minute of exercise)

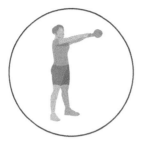

1. KETTLEBELL OR DUMBBELL SWING, PAGE 28

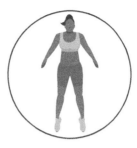

2. X-JUMP, PAGE 55

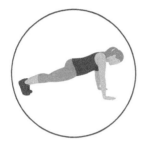

3. PLANK JACK, PAGE 32

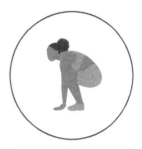

4. BURPEE, PAGE 21

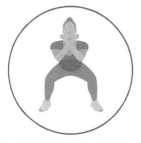

5. SQUAT JUMP , PAGE 44

Power Legs Workout

Here's another cardio-focused workout, offering lots of bang for your buck.

 # OF CIRCUITS X DURATION 3 rounds, 1 minute of exercise (40 seconds of work, 20 seconds of rest)

TOTAL WORKOUT TIME 15 minutes

TOTAL TIME 25 minutes, including warm-up, workout, and cool down

WARM-UP 5 minutes with a quick functional circuit or moderate cardio of choice

RECOVERY 30 seconds, if needed, before moving on to the next round

COOL DOWN 5 minutes (page 56)

COMMON MISTAKES AND HOW TO AVOID THEM Set yourself up for proper form and move efficiently. For safety, move a little more slowly with great form rather than going too fast.

CHANGE IT UP To reduce impact, eliminate the jumps. You can still get an awesome workout and keep at least one foot on the floor at all times.

Strength and HIIT Workout (3 rounds, 1 minute of exercise [40 seconds work, 20 seconds rest])

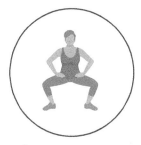

1. PLIÉ SQUAT JUMP, PAGE 34

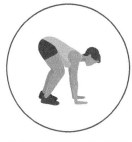

2. THRUSTER, PAGE 49

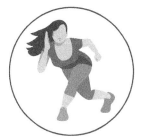

3. SKATER, PAGE 42

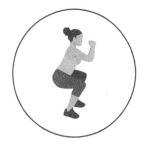

4. ROTATING SQUAT JUMP, PAGE 38

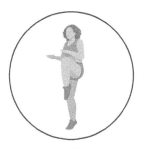

5. HIGH KNEES , PAGE 24

Leg Burn and Blast

This workout combines strength moves with explosive power exercises. Burn a high number of calories in a short time while getting the benefits of both strength and cardio. All you need is your own body weight.

 # OF CIRCUITS X DURATION 3 rounds, 1 minute per exercise

TOTAL WORKOUT TIME 15 minutes

TOTAL TIME 25 minutes, including warm-up, workout, and cool down

WARM-UP 5 minutes with a quick functional circuit or moderate cardio of choice

RECOVERY 30 seconds to 3 minutes, if needed, before moving on to the next round

COOL DOWN 5 minutes (page 56)

COMMON MISTAKES AND HOW TO AVOID THEM A minute can feel like forever. Work as long as you can, take a few minutes to breathe and rest, then hop back into it. Over time, you'll be able to complete more of each minute-long segment.

REMEMBER If you don't have a resistance band, that's okay—complete the movements without them.

CHANGE IT UP For the plank jacks, try them with your hands on a wall or a countertop. To decrease the intensity, try curtsy lunges (page 42) instead of the skater and ditch the resistance bands. To make the movements more challenging, hold a weight at your chest for the wall sit and two weights for the sit squat.

Strength and HIIT Workout (3 rounds, 1 minute per exercise)

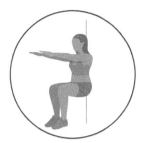

1. WALL SIT, PAGE 53

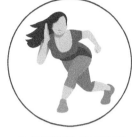

2. SKATER, PAGE 42

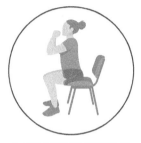

3. SIT SQUAT, PAGE 41

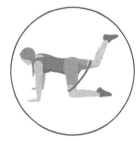

4. RESISTANCE BAND DONKEY KICK, PAGE 36, (ALTERNATE SIDES)

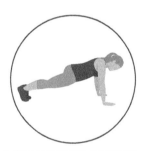

5. PLANK JACK, PAGE 32

Lower Body Power AMRAP

This workout consists of strength movements with less of an emphasis on cardio. Feel free to complete this one the day before or after an arms HIIT or pure HIIT workout.

 # OF CIRCUITS X DURATION This workout is meant to be completed AMRAP style, as many rounds as possible in 15 minutes. Set a timer and work through each round.

TOTAL WORKOUT TIME 15 minutes

TOTAL TIME 25 minutes, including warm-up, workout, and cool down

WARM-UP 5 minutes with a quick functional circuit or moderate cardio of choice

RECOVERY 30 seconds to 1 minute, if needed, before moving on to the next round

COOL DOWN 5 minutes (page 56)

COMMON MISTAKES AND HOW TO AVOID THEM Always start off with a slightly lighter weight than you think you'll need. If you can execute the movements with great form and you're not feeling challenged, add in more weight. It's better to start off too light than too heavy.

CHANGE IT UP To decrease the intensity, perform the exercises without additional weight. For more of a challenge, hold heavier weights.

Strength Circuit (AMRAP, 15 minutes)

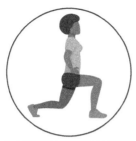

1. ALTERNATING LUNGE, PAGE 17, X 12 REPS

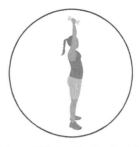

2. SQUAT TO OVERHEAD PRESS, PAGE 45, X 10 REPS

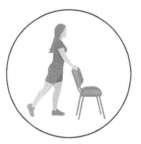

3. HIP EXTENSION, PAGE 25 X 10 REPS

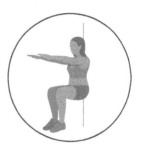

4. WALL SIT, PAGE 53, X 30 SECONDS

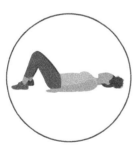

5. HIP RAISE, PAGE 26, X 15 REPS

Squat Burner Workout

This workout includes variations of one of my very favorite exercises: the squat, which works your quads, hamstrings, glutes, and core.

 # OF CIRCUITS X DURATION 3 rounds, 1 minute per exercise

TOTAL WORKOUT TIME 15 minutes

TOTAL TIME 25 minutes, including warm-up, workout, and cool down

WARM-UP 5 minutes with a quick functional circuit or moderate cardio of choice

RECOVERY 30 seconds, if needed, before moving on to the next round

COOL DOWN 5 minutes (page 56)

COMMON MISTAKES AND HOW TO AVOID THEM Sit down and back for your squat, as if you were moving into an imaginary chair. Keep your knees stacked over your ankles, core tight, and shoulders relaxed. Try to maintain a neutral back instead of tucking the hips or arching.

CHANGE IT UP To decrease the intensity, perform the movements for 30 seconds instead of 1 minute. Gradually add time as you get stronger. To decrease the impact of the squat jumps, perform bodyweight squats (page 44) instead. To make the workout more challenging, hold a heavier weight for the strength exercises.

Squat Burner Circuit (3 rounds, 1 minute per exercise)

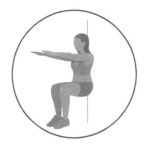

1. WALL SIT, PAGE 53

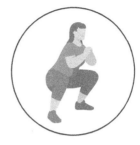

2. SUMO SQUAT, PAGE 47

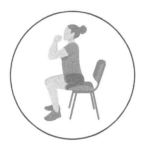

3. SIT SQUAT, PAGE 41

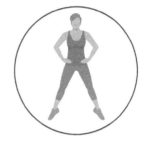

4. PLIÉ SQUAT JUMP, PAGE 34

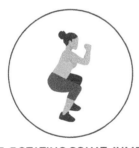

5. ROTATING SQUAT JUMP, PAGE 38, (30 SECONDS)

Baby Got Booty Workout

This workout includes all my go-to exercises for building strong, lean glutes and legs. We'll do a superset of two similar exercises (first the squats and then the lunge, step-up, and X-jump) and complete a cardio blast before moving on to the next round.

 # OF CIRCUITS X DURATION 3 mini circuits, 5 minutes each

TOTAL WORKOUT TIME 15 minutes

TOTAL TIME 25 minutes, including warm-up, workout, and cool down

WARM-UP 5 minutes with a quick functional circuit or moderate cardio of choice

RECOVERY 30 seconds, if needed, before moving on to the next round

COOL DOWN 5 minutes (page 56)

COMMON MISTAKES AND HOW TO AVOID THEM For the donkey kick, move from your glutes and hamstrings not the arch of your back. Keep your back flat, spine long, and both hips parallel to the floor. Pull in your core and exhale as you lift your leg.

REMEMBER You can always add in some steady state cardio after your workout if you have more time, even if it's just 10 minutes spent walking around the block to cool down and shake your legs out.

CHANGE IT UP For the mountain climbers, place your hands on a wall or a countertop. To decrease the intensity, perform bodyweight squats (page 44) instead of the squat jumps and walk your feet out and in for the X-jumps (instead of jumping). To make things more challenging, hold heavier weights for any or all of the sit squats, lunges, or step-ups.

Mini Circuit 1 (5 minutes)

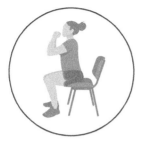

**1. SIT SQUAT, PAGE 41,
X 10 REPS**

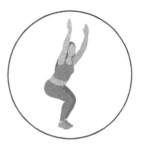

**2. CLOSE SQUAT, PAGE 22,
X 10 REPS**

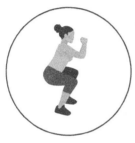

**3. ROTATING SQUAT JUMP,
PAGE 38, X 10 REPS**

Mini Circuit 2 (5 minutes)

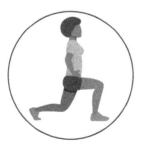

**1. ALTERNATING LUNGE,
PAGE 17, X 12 REPS**

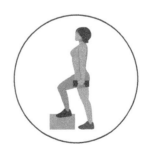

2. STEP-UP, PAGE 46, X 20 REPS

CONTINUED

Baby Got Booty Workout CONTINUED

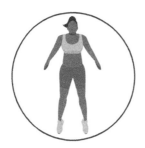

3. X-JUMP, PAGE 55, X 20 REPS

Mini Circuit 3 (5 minutes)

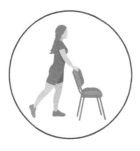

**1. HIP EXTENSION,
PAGE 25, X 20 REPS**

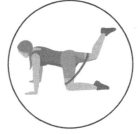

**2. RESISTANCE BAND DONKEY
KICK, PAGE 36, X 20 REPS**

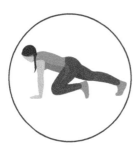

**3. MOUNTAIN CLIMBER,
PAGE 30, X 40 REPS**

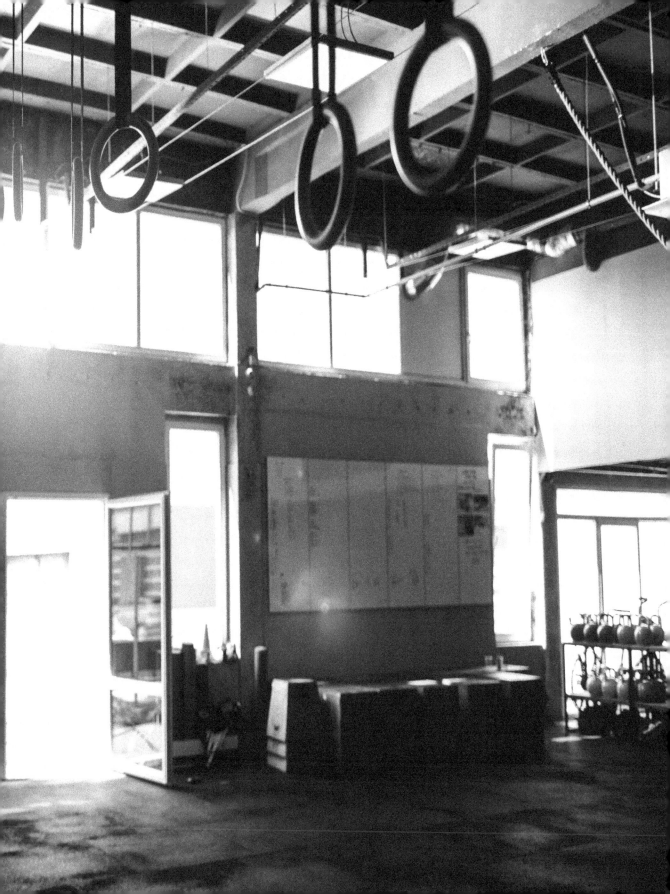

HIIT the Limit Legs Workout

This incredibly challenging HIIT workout for the legs focuses on 45-second rounds and 15 seconds of rest for 15 exercises. Pace yourself, and remember you can always switch to the low-impact variation—just keep moving!

 # OF CIRCUITS X DURATION 1 round of 15 exercises. Work 45 seconds per exercise with a 15-second rest in between.

TOTAL WORKOUT TIME 15 minutes

TOTAL TIME 25 minutes, including warm-up, workout, and cool down

WARM-UP 5 minutes with a quick functional circuit or moderate cardio of choice

RECOVERY 1 minute before starting your cool down

COOL DOWN 5 minutes (page 56)

COMMON MISTAKES AND HOW TO AVOID THEM Don't overdo it on the first try. Start with the low-impact variations of the exercises, and add in some of the high-impact and jumping variations when you're comfortable.

CHANGE IT UP To decrease the intensity, perform the movements for 30 seconds instead of 45 seconds. To decrease the impact of the squat jumps, do bodyweight squats (page 44) instead. You can always eliminate the jumps to dial down the impact and intensity. To make the workout more challenging, hold a weight for any or all of the step-ups, sumo squats, lunges, reverse lunges, wall sits, or sit squats.

Strength and Cardio Workout
(45 seconds work, 15 seconds rest per exercise)

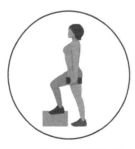

1. STEP-UP, PAGE 46

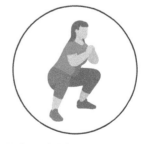

2. SUMO SQUAT, PAGE 47

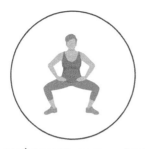

3. PLIÉ SQUAT JUMP, PAGE 34

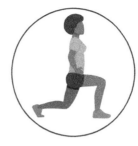

4. ALTERNATING LUNGE, PAGE 17

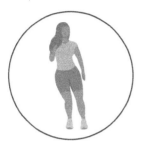

5. SKI HOP, PAGE 43

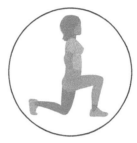

6. REVERSE LUNGE, PAGE 37

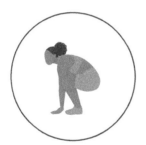

7. BURPEE, PAGE 21

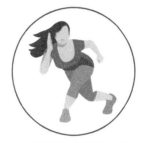

8. SKATER, PAGE 42

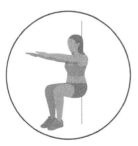

9. WALL SIT, PAGE 53

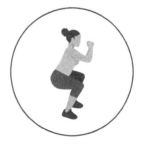

10. ROTATING SQUAT JUMP, PAGE 38

CONTINUED

HIIT the Limit Legs Workout CONTINUED

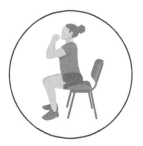

11. SIT SQUAT, PAGE 41

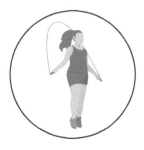

12. JUMP ROPE, PAGE 27

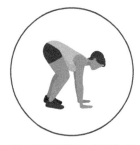

13. THRUSTER, PAGE 49

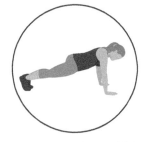

14. PLANK JACK, PAGE 32

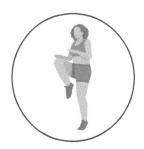

15. HIGH KNEES, PAGE 24

Full Body

Total body workouts give you the most bang for your buck. You're able to strengthen and work multiple muscle groups at once—the best kind of multitasking—often resulting in a higher calorie-burn. If you can only exercise once or twice a week, this is the best use of your time.

Total body workouts can be completed anywhere, including the park, gym, your bedroom, or the backyard—the possibilities are endless.

The Whole Package Strength Workout

This workout focuses on pure strength for the entire body and is an excellent workout to do the day after a tough cardio-driven HIIT or an easier steady state cardio session. If you find you have more time, follow up with a pure HIIT or cardio workout.

 # OF CIRCUITS X DURATION 3 sets of 12 reps per exercise

TOTAL WORKOUT TIME About 15 minutes

TOTAL TIME 20 to 25 minutes, including warm-up, workout, and cool down

WARM-UP 5 minutes, moderate cardio of choice

RECOVERY 30 seconds, if needed, before moving on to the next round

COOL DOWN 5 minutes (page 56)

COMMON MISTAKES AND HOW TO AVOID THEM Don't move too quickly through the exercises. Take time for proper form and to breathe.

CHANGE IT UP To modify, use lighter weights. You can also modify the push-ups by placing your hands on a wall or a countertop. For a more advanced variation, hold heavier weights.

HIIT Circuit (3 sets of 12 reps per exercise)

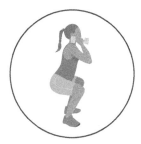

1. SQUAT TO OVERHEAD PRESS, PAGE 45

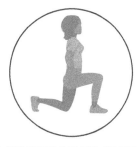

2. REVERSE LUNGE, PAGE 37

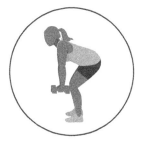

3. BENT-OVER ROW, PAGE 18

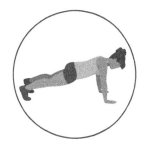

4. PUSH-UP, PAGE 35

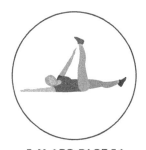

5. X-ABS, PAGE 54

Total Body Strength + HIIT

This workout combines strength exercises with HIIT blasts for a short and sweaty workout.

 # OF CIRCUITS X DURATION 3 mini circuits, 5 minutes each

TOTAL WORKOUT TIME 15 minutes

TOTAL TIME 20 to 25 minutes, including warm-up, workout, and cool down

WARM-UP 5 minutes, moderate cardio of choice

RECOVERY 30 seconds, if needed, before moving on to the next round

COOL DOWN 5 minutes (page 56)

COMMON MISTAKES AND HOW TO AVOID THEM For the kettlebell and dumbbell swings, people often use their arms for the movement. Instead, use the power of your glutes and core to swing the dumbbell or kettlebell. The arms are just there to hold on to the weight, not to do the work.

CHANGE IT UP To lessen the intensity, eliminate the jumps, walking your feet back to plank for the burpee, and walking your feet out and in instead of hopping for the plank jacks. For a more advanced variation, hold heavier weights.

HIIT Circuit 1 (5 minutes)

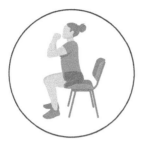

1. SIT SQUAT, PAGE 41, X 12 REPS

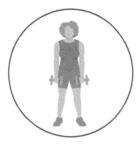

2. UPRIGHT ROW, PAGE 52, X 12 REPS

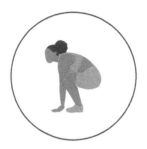

3. BURPEE, PAGE 21, X 10 REPS

HIIT Circuit 2 (5 minutes)

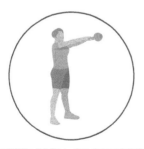

1. KETTLEBELL OR DUMBBELL SWING, PAGE 28, X 15 REPS

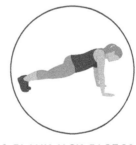

2. PLANK JACK, PAGE 32, X 15 REPS

CONTINUED

Total Body Strength + HIIT CONTINUED

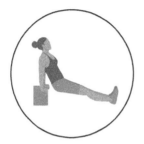

**3. TRICEPS DIP, PAGE 50,
X 10 REPS**

Mini Circuit 3 (5 minutes)

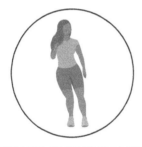

1. SKI HOP, PAGE 43, X 20 REPS

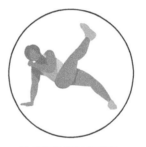

**2. BREAKDANCER,
PAGE 20, X 20 REPS**

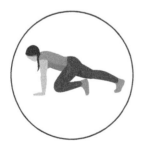

**3. MOUNTAIN CLIMBER,
PAGE 30, X 20 REPS**

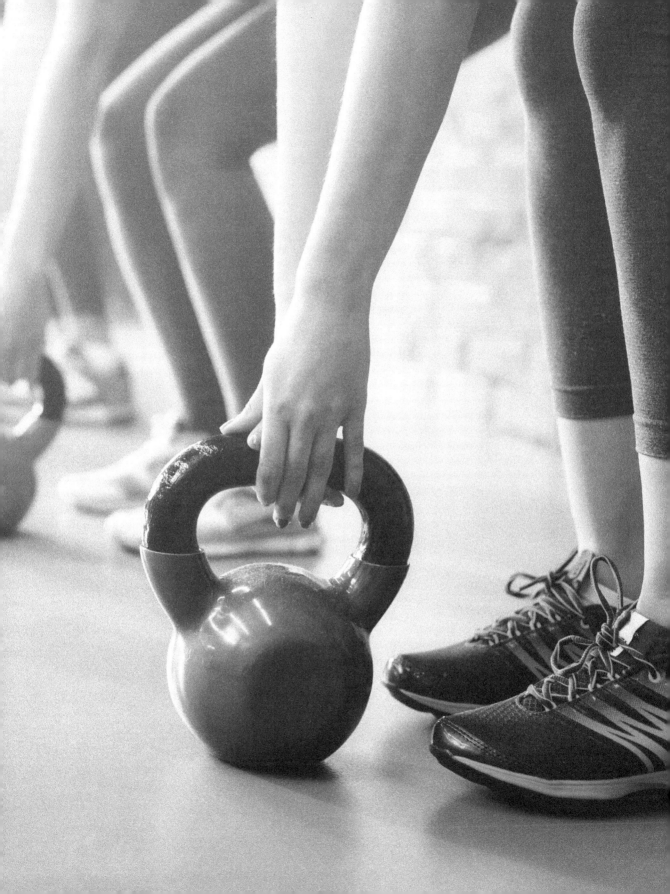

Burpee Buy-in

This workout includes a burpee buy-in. Before beginning the actual workout circuit, complete 25 burpees. Doing so will get your heart rate up and challenge your entire body before the circuit.

 # OF CIRCUITS X DURATION This workout is meant to be completed AMRAP style, as many rounds as possible in 15 minutes. Set a timer and work through each round.

TOTAL WORKOUT TIME 15 minutes (5 minutes for burpees, 10 minutes for the circuit)

TOTAL TIME 20 to 25 minutes, including warm-up, workout, and cool down

WARM-UP 5 minutes, moderate cardio of choice

RECOVERY 30 seconds to 1 minute between rounds

COOL DOWN 5 minutes (page 56)

COMMON MISTAKES AND HOW TO AVOID THEM Watch your form on the burpees. The tendency can be to rush, not "hopping" your feet back uniformly until your back is flat (like the push-up position). Take your time and focus on the movements to avoid injury.

CHANGE IT UP Modify the burpee by eliminating the jump, placing your hands on a wall instead of the floor, or both. To decrease the intensity, hold lighter weights. For a more advanced variation, add a tuck jump (raising your knees to your chest as you spring up) at the top of each burpee, or a push-up once you're in the plank position at the completion of the exercise. Increase the intensity by holding heavier weights for any or all of the sit squats, biceps curls, or triceps extensions.

Burpee Circuit (5 minutes, AMRAP)

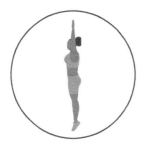

1. BURPEE, PAGE 21, X 25 REPS

HIIT Circuit (AMRAP, 10 minutes)

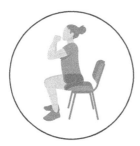

1. SIT SQUAT, PAGE 41, X 10 REPS

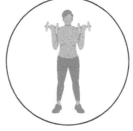

2. BICEPS CURL, PAGE 19, X 10 REPS

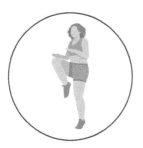

3. HIGH KNEES, PAGE 24, X 30 REPS

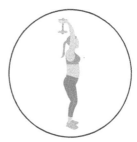

4. TRICEPS EXTENSION, PAGE 51, X 10 REPS

Plank and Power Burner

This workout includes a plank variation at the end of each circuit, challenging your core and stability to support proper posture and good alignment.

 # OF CIRCUITS X DURATION This workout is meant to be completed AMRAP style, as many rounds as possible in 15 minutes. Set a timer and work through each circuit. For round 2, substitute plank jacks for a 30-second plank. For round 3, substitute plank jacks for a side plank, 15 seconds each side. Keep switching it up for subsequent rounds.

TOTAL WORKOUT TIME 15 minutes

TOTAL TIME 25 minutes, including warm-up, workout, and cool down

WARM-UP 5 minutes, moderate cardio of choice

RECOVERY 30 seconds, if needed

COOL DOWN 5 minutes (page 56)

COMMON MISTAKES AND HOW TO AVOID THEM Avoid letting your hips drop, arching your back, or hiking your hips into the air. Aim to be as straight as possible, breathe, and keep your belly pulled up and in.

REMEMBER You get to do a different plank variation at the end of each round, so switch it up and use any variations you love.

CHANGE IT UP For the push-up, place your hands on a wall or a countertop. For the plank jacks, walk your feet out and in, instead of hopping. To decrease the intensity, modify the squat jumps to bodyweight squats (page 44). To make this workout more challenging, hold heavier weights.

HIIT Circuit (AMRAP, 15 minutes)

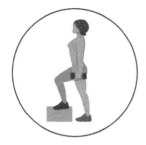

1. STEP-UP, PAGE 46, X 10 REPS EACH SIDE LEG

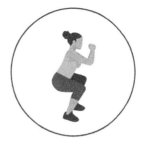

2. ROTATING SQUAT JUMP, PAGE 38, X 20 REPS TOTAL

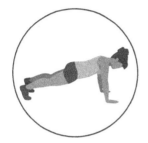

3. PUSH-UP, PAGE 35, X 10 REPS

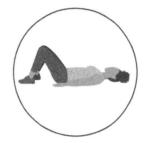

4. HIP RAISE, PAGE 26, X 15 REPS

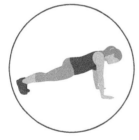

5. PLANK JACK, PAGE 32, X 15 REPS

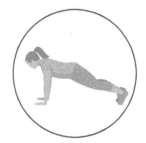

ROUND 2: END WITH PLANK, PAGE 31, X 30 SECONDS

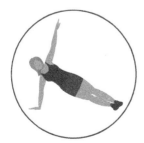

ROUND 3: END WITH SIDE PLANK, PAGE 40, X 15 SECONDS EACH SIDE

Total Body HIIT Challenge

This workout includes strength training exercises that will get your heart rate up. This is a great way to HIIT train while getting a solid strength workout.

 # OF CIRCUITS X DURATION 3 rounds, 45 seconds of work and 15 seconds of rest (1 minute per exercise)

TOTAL WORKOUT TIME 15 minutes

TOTAL TIME 25 minutes, including warm-up, workout, and cool down

WARM-UP 5 minutes, moderate cardio

RECOVERY 30 seconds, if needed

COOL DOWN 5 minutes (page 56)

COMMON MISTAKES AND HOW TO AVOID THEM For the donkey kick, align your knees under your hips and place your hands under your shoulders. Keep your hips parallel to the ground and your neck long. Use your glutes to lift your leg instead of relying on momentum and keep your back flat.

REMEMBER Lunges should be 90-degree angles in the front and back legs.

CHANGE IT UP To modify the push-up to side plank, perform this move on your knees, and as you rotate to side plank, keep your bottom knee on the ground (extending your top leg). To decrease the intensity, take away the resistance band for the donkey kick. To make this workout more challenging, use heavier weights.

HIIT with Weights Circuit (3 rounds, 1 minute per exercise)

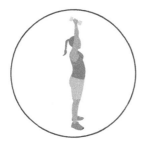

1. SQUAT TO OVERHEAD PRESS, PAGE 45

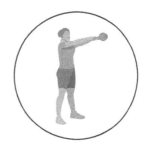

2. KETTLEBELL OR DUMBBELL SWING, PAGE 28

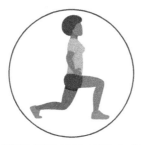

3. ALTERNATING LUNGE, PAGE 17

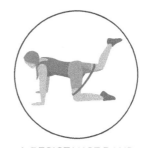

4. RESISTANCE BAND DONKEY KICK, PAGE 36

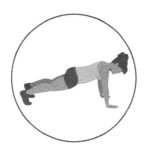

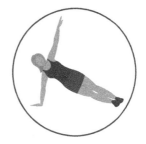

5. PUSH-UP, PAGE 35, TO SIDE PLANK, PAGE 40, (ALTERNATE SIDES)

Off to the Races—
Pure Cardio

This workout is pure cardio HIIT! Ideal the day after or before a more challenging strength day, this one should only be done one to two times per week on non-consecutive days. This is classic HIIT at its best—a sweaty combination of total body moves that will elevate your metabolism and help improve speed and power.

 # OF CIRCUITS X DURATION 3 rounds, 1 minute per exercise (30 seconds of work and 30 seconds of rest)

TOTAL WORKOUT TIME 15 minutes

TOTAL TIME 25 minutes, including warm-up, workout, and cool down

WARM-UP 5 minutes, moderate cardio of choice

RECOVERY 30 seconds, if needed

COOL DOWN 5 minutes (page 56)

COMMON MISTAKES AND HOW TO AVOID THEM Move for the entire 30-second block, even if you need to modify the exercises or intensity.

CHANGE IT UP To reduce impact, move more slowly and deliberately and eliminate the jumps. For the rotating squat jumps, walk to each side and squat. Use curtsy lunges (page 42) instead of the skaters. To make this workout more challenging, move quickly and more dynamically. Try to get as much height as possible for the jumps.

HIIT Circuit (3 rounds, 1 minute per exercise)

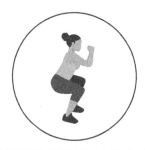

1. ROTATING SQUAT JUMP, PAGE 38

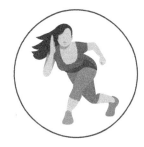

2. SKATER, PAGE 42

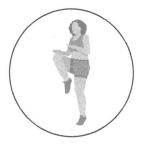

3. HIGH KNEES, PAGE 24

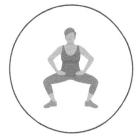

4. PLIÉ SQUAT JUMP, PAGE 34

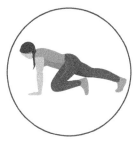

5. MOUNTAIN CLIMBER, PAGE 30

Sprint It to Win It

Here's another cardio-heavy HIIT workout for either the day before or after a strength training day. (You shouldn't do a workout like this more than one to two times per week on non-consecutive days.) The combination of exercises helps boost metabolism, power, and speed.

 # OF CIRCUITS X DURATION 3 rounds, 1 minute per exercise (45 seconds of work and 15 seconds of rest)

TOTAL WORKOUT TIME 15 minutes

TOTAL TIME 25 minutes, including warm-up, workout, and cool down

WARM-UP 5 minutes, moderate cardio of choice

RECOVERY 30 seconds, if needed

COOL DOWN 5 minutes (page 56)

COMMON MISTAKES AND HOW TO AVOID THEM Any time you jump, land with soft knees and avoid locking the knee joint.

CHANGE IT UP If you don't have a jump rope, perform faux jump rope, pretending you're jumping (without the rope!), or jog or march in place. To reduce impact, do regular plié squats without the jumps and walk, not hop, your feet back to plank in the thrusters. Moving more quickly through each exercise while emphasizing each movement will make the workout more challenging.

HIIT Circuit (3 rounds, 1 minute per exercise)

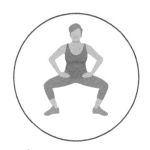

1. PLIÉ SQUAT JUMP, PAGE 34

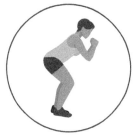

2. THRUSTER, PAGE 49

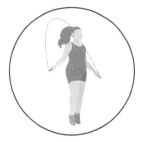

3. JUMP ROPE, PAGE 27

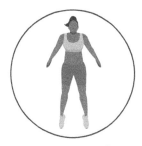

4. X-JUMP, PAGE 55

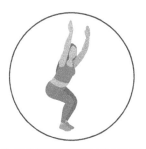

5. CLOSE SQUAT, PAGE 22

Total Body Tabata (1 Tabata Round)

This is our first workout using Tabata intervals, a type of training modeled after the findings of a well-known study by Dr. Izumi Tabata. He compared two groups of exercisers, one doing steady-state workouts and another doing interval workouts. The latter achieved the same weight loss and fitness improvement of the former but in a quarter of the time.

Here's the Tabata formula:

8 rounds: 20 seconds of hard work + 10 seconds rest = 4 minutes

For this workout, you'll complete 8 minutes of strength, then one 4-minute Tabata interval set.

 # OF CIRCUITS X DURATION 2 rounds strength: 1 minute per each of 4 exercises = 8 minutes; 1 Tabata interval set = 4 minutes (8 rounds: 20 seconds of work and 10 seconds of rest per each of 4 exercises)

TOTAL WORKOUT TIME 12 minutes

TOTAL TIME 22 minutes, including warm-up, workout, and cool down

WARM-UP 5 minutes, moderate cardio of choice

RECOVERY 1 minute, if needed, before starting the Tabata round

COOL DOWN 5 minutes (page 56)

COMMON MISTAKES AND HOW TO AVOID THEM For the hip extension, keep both hips facing forward. For the Tabata round, work as hard as possible. You're only going strong for 20 seconds at a time so you can ramp up the intensity!

CHANGE IT UP For the mountain climbers, place your hands on a wall or a countertop. To reduce impact, hold light weights (or no weights) for the strength circuit and eliminate the jump on the Tabata rounds. Jog or march in place for the high knees. Squat instead of doing the ski hops. Modify the burpees by placing your hand on a wall and ditching the jumps. To make this workout more challenging, hold heavier weights for the strength circuit or make each movement more pronounced.

Strength Circuit (2 rounds, 1 minute per exercise)

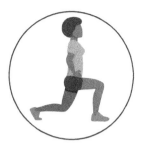

1. ALTERNATING LUNGE TO PAUSE, PAGE 17

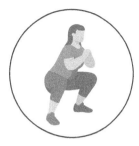

2. SUMO SQUAT, PAGE 47

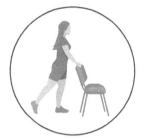

3. HIP EXTENSION, PAGE 25

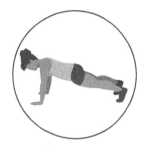

4. PUSH-UP, PAGE 35

Tabata (20 seconds on, 10 seconds off for each exercise; 4 minutes total)

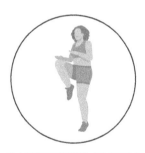

1. HIGH KNEES, PAGE 24

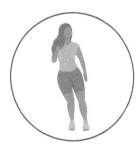

2. SKI HOP, PAGE 43

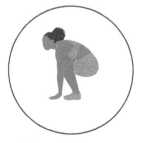

3. BURPEE, PAGE 21

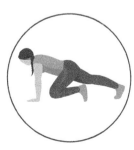

4. MOUNTAIN CLIMBER, PAGE 30

Total Body Tabata (2 Tabata Rounds)

This workout includes two Tabata rounds for an even sweatier workout challenge than the previous one. Here, you'll complete 4 minutes of strength, capped off with two 4-minute Tabata rounds.

 # OF CIRCUITS X DURATION 1 round strength: 1 minute per each of 4 exercises = 4 minutes; 2 Tabata interval sets = 8 minutes (16 rounds: 20 seconds of work and 10 seconds of rest per each of 4 exercises)

TOTAL WORKOUT TIME 12 minutes

TOTAL TIME 22 minutes, including warm-up, workout, and cool down

WARM-UP 5 minutes, moderate cardio of choice

RECOVERY 1 minute, if needed, before starting the Tabata round

COOL DOWN 5 minutes (page 56)

COMMON MISTAKES AND HOW TO AVOID THEM For the breakdancer, maintain your breathing and keep your core up and in to support your low back.

CHANGE IT UP To reduce impact, use lighter weights (or no weights) and forgo the jump on the Tabata rounds. Try curtsy lunges (page 42) instead of the skaters, bodyweight squats (page 44) instead of the squat jumps, place your hands on a wall for mountain climbers, and try walking instead of jumping for the burpees, thrusters, and X-jumps. For more of a challenge, emphasize the form of the movements and use heavier weights.

Strength Circuit (1 round , 4 minutes)

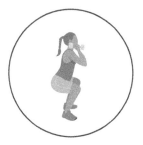

1. SQUAT TO OVERHEAD PRESS, PAGE 45

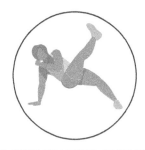

2. BREAKDANCER, PAGE 20

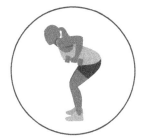

3. BENT-OVER ROW, PAGE 18

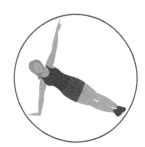

4. SIDE PLANK, PAGE 40, (30 SECONDS EACH SIDE)

Tabata 1 (20 seconds on, 10 seconds off for each exercise; 4 minutes total)

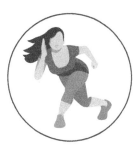

1. SKATER, PAGE 42

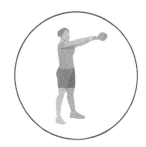

2. KETTLEBELL OR DUMBBELL SWING, PAGE 28

CONTINUED

Total Body Tabata (2 Tabata Rounds) CONTINUED

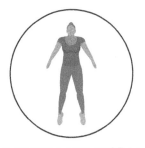

3. SQUAT JUMP , PAGE 44

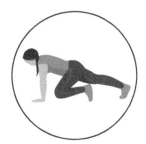

4. PUSH-UP, PAGE 35

Tabata 2 (20 seconds on, 10 seconds off for each exercise; 4 minutes total)

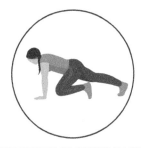

1. MOUNTAIN CLIMBER, PAGE 30

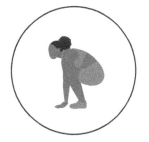

2. BURPEE, PAGE 21

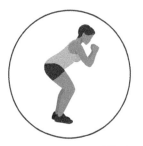

3. THRUSTER, PAGE 49

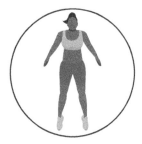

4. X-JUMP, PAGE 55

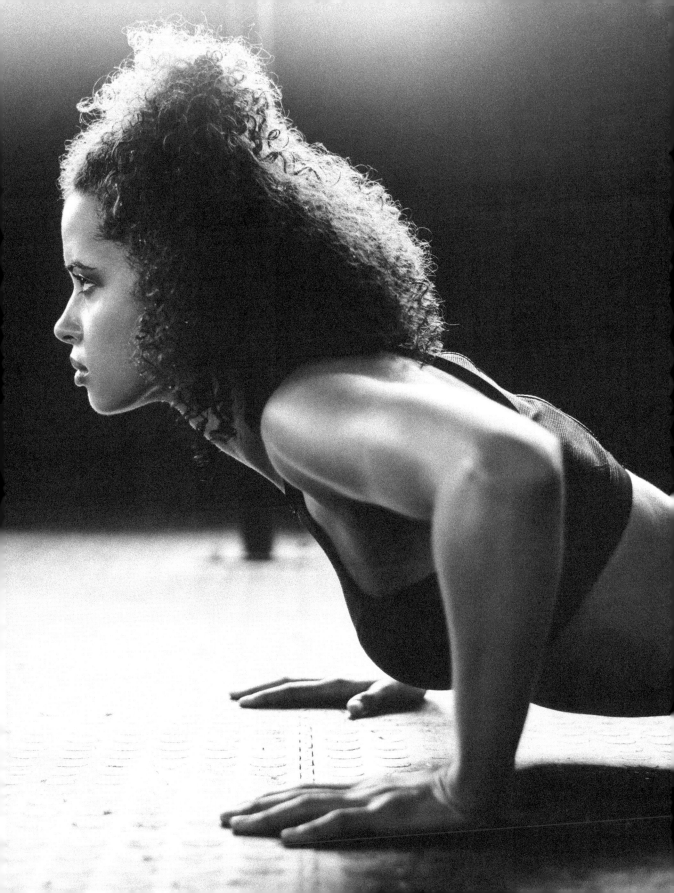

Total Body Tabata (3 Tabata Rounds)

Now we've reached the most challenging workout in this book—the three 4-minute Tabata rounds back to back!

 # OF CIRCUITS X DURATION 3 Tabata interval sets (24 rounds total: 20 seconds of work and 10 seconds of rest per each of 4 exercises in each set)

TOTAL WORKOUT TIME 12 minutes

TOTAL TIME 22 minutes, including warm-up, workout, and cool down

WARM-UP 5 minutes, moderate cardio of choice

RECOVERY 1 minute after the sets

COOL DOWN 5 minutes (page 56)

COMMON MISTAKES AND HOW TO AVOID THEM Move as quickly as possible to increase your heart rate.

CHANGE IT UP Eliminating the jump on the Tabata rounds will make the workout more low-impact. Try curtsy lunges (page 42) instead of skaters, bodyweight squats instead of squat jumps, place your hands on a wall for mountain climbers, and try walking instead of jumping for the burpees, thrusters, and X-jumps. If you want to make this already challenging workout even more so, emphasize each movement—for example, jumping as high as possible or squatting as low as you can—will do the trick.

Tabata 1 (20 seconds on, 10 off for each exercise; 4 minutes total)

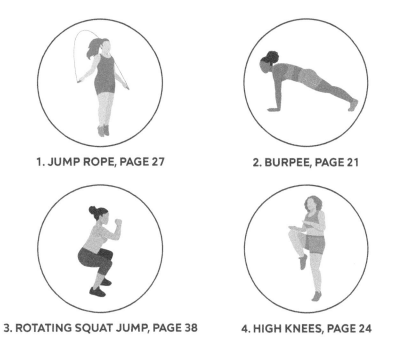

1. JUMP ROPE, PAGE 27

2. BURPEE, PAGE 21

3. ROTATING SQUAT JUMP, PAGE 38

4. HIGH KNEES, PAGE 24

Tabata 2 (20 seconds on, 10 off for each exercise; 4 minutes total)

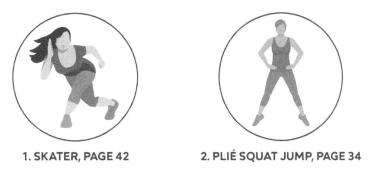

1. SKATER, PAGE 42

2. PLIÉ SQUAT JUMP, PAGE 34

CONTINUED

Total Body Tabata (3 Tabata Rounds) CONTINUED

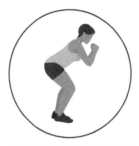

3. THRUSTER, PAGE 49

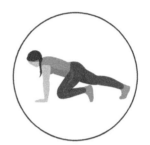

4. MOUNTAIN CLIMBER, PAGE 30

Tabata 3 (20 seconds on, 10 off for each exercise; 4 minutes total)

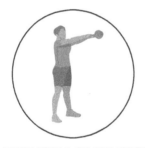

**1. KETTLEBELL OR DUMBBELL
SWING, PAGE 28**

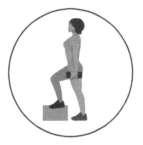

2. STEP-UP, PAGE 46

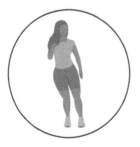

3. SKI HOP, PAGE 43

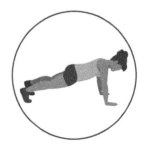

4. PUSH-UP, PAGE 35

THE SCIENCE BEHIND RECOVERY

Recovery is just as important as the work. When you enjoy exercising, it might be tricky to convince yourself to take a day off. But those recovery days are when the magic happens. When we work out, we create tiny tears in our muscle fibers. When the muscle repairs itself during recovery, those tears heal themselves and also become strong. This is what improves the density of our muscle tissue over time. When we exercise, the body uses glycogen (stored carbohydrates) to fuel our activity. Recovery allows those stores to replenish.

If you continue to exercise without adequate time for recovery, you can feel rundown, unnaturally sore, and fatigued. You may experience immune issues and an elevated heart rate, all symptoms of overtraining. Your body needs at least one to two full days of rest each week to replenish and recover to get stronger. Without proper rest each week, you're also more susceptible to injury from overuse.

What should you do on your recovery days? Take a leisurely walk outside, enjoy a long stretching session, go to a restorative yoga class, get a massage, take a nap—do the things that make you feel relaxed and restored. Massage, compression, and active recovery have all been shown to help reduce muscle soreness and perceived fatigue. Know that by taking this time to encourage recovery, you'll be able to hit your workouts stronger next time!

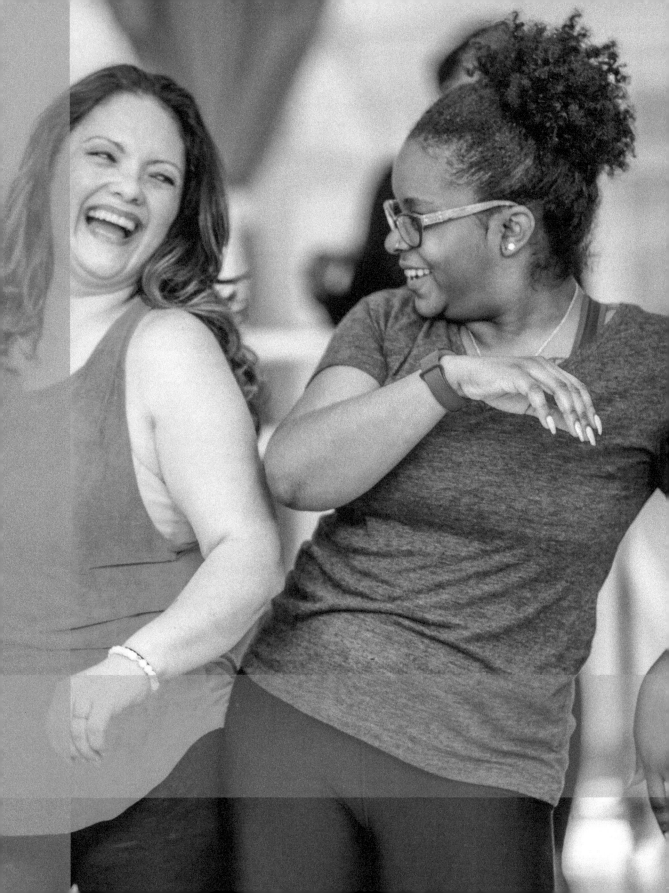

CHAPTER FOUR
Track Your Progress

The fitness tracker in this chapter is a great tool to track your progress as you complete your workouts and go after your health and fitness goals. Tracking can be extremely beneficial because you can see how you progress over time, such as by lifting heavier weights, completing more rounds of an AMRAP workout, or maintaining consistency. It can be so motivating to look back and see what you've accomplished.

This fitness tracker will give you an overview of your achievements over the long term and also help you determine patterns for mood and sleep. When you look back at your tracked progress in four-week blocks, you may be surprised by how much you've improved, even if at the time you hadn't felt like you were making huge strides.

Use this tool to track your daily workouts in addition to other critical factors in your health and well-being, like water intake, fresh produce consumption, mood, and sleep quality (did you sleep soundly or were you restless?). At the top, you'll see "This Week's Goals," where you can also write a mantra, a motivational quote, or something you want to keep in mind. I like to use this space to write something that makes me grateful. By maintaining an attitude of thankfulness and gratitude, I'm more likely to be easy on myself and share patience and love with others, which positively affects my mood. You can find more pages for download at **callistomediabooks.com/15minutehiitforwomen**.

Weekly Fitness Journal

THIS WEEK'S GOALS:

1) _____

2) _____

3) _____

Check off daily intake of: Water 🥛 Fruit 🍎 Greens/veggies 🌿

SUNDAY

☐ Core and Abs | ☐ Legs and Glutes | ☐ Full Body
I feel: 😊 😐 🙁
Sleep quantity and quality: _____
Workout notes: _____

MONDAY

☐ Core and Abs | ☐ Legs and Glutes | ☐ Full Body
I feel: 😊 😐 🙁
Sleep quantity and quality: _____
Workout notes: _____

TUESDAY

☐ Core and Abs | ☐ Legs and Glutes | ☐ Full Body
I feel: 😊 😐 🙁
Sleep quantity and quality: _____
Workout notes: _____

WEDNESDAY

☐☐☐☐☐☐☐☐ 🍎🍎 🌿🌿🌿🌿

☐ Core and Abs | ☐ Legs and Glutes | ☐ Full Body

I feel: 😊 😐 😟

Sleep quantity and quality: _____

Workout notes: _____

THURSDAY

☐☐☐☐☐☐☐☐ 🍎🍎 🌿🌿🌿🌿

☐ Core and Abs | ☐ Legs and Glutes | ☐ Full Body

I feel: 😊 😐 😟

Sleep quantity and quality: _____

Workout notes: _____

FRIDAY

☐☐☐☐☐☐☐☐ 🍎🍎 🌿🌿🌿🌿

☐ Core and Abs | ☐ Legs and Glutes | ☐ Full Body

I feel: 😊 😐 😟

Sleep quantity and quality: _____

Workout notes: _____

SATURDAY

☐☐☐☐☐☐☐☐ 🍎🍎 🌿🌿🌿🌿

☐ Core and Abs | ☐ Legs and Glutes | ☐ Full Body

I feel: 😊 😐 😟

Sleep quantity and quality: _____

Workout notes: _____

Weekly Fitness Journal

THIS WEEK'S GOALS:

1) _____

2) _____

3) _____

Check off daily intake of: Water 🥛 Fruit 🍎 Greens/veggies 🌿

SUNDAY

🥛🥛🥛🥛🥛🥛🥛🥛 🍎🍎 🌿🌿🌿🌿

☐ Core and Abs | ☐ Legs and Glutes | ☐ Full Body

I feel: 😊 😐 ☹️

Sleep quantity and quality: _____

Workout notes: _____

MONDAY

🥛🥛🥛🥛🥛🥛🥛🥛 🍎🍎 🌿🌿🌿🌿

☐ Core and Abs | ☐ Legs and Glutes | ☐ Full Body

I feel: 😊 😐 ☹️

Sleep quantity and quality: _____

Workout notes: _____

TUESDAY

🥛🥛🥛🥛🥛🥛🥛🥛 🍎🍎 🌿🌿🌿🌿

☐ Core and Abs | ☐ Legs and Glutes | ☐ Full Body

I feel: 😊 😐 ☹️

Sleep quantity and quality: _____

Workout notes: _____

WEDNESDAY

□□□□□□□□ 🍎🍎 🌿🌿🌿🌿

☐ Core and Abs | ☐ Legs and Glutes | ☐ Full Body

I feel: 😊 😐 🙁

Sleep quantity and quality: _____

Workout notes: _____

THURSDAY

□□□□□□□□ 🍎🍎 🌿🌿🌿🌿

☐ Core and Abs | ☐ Legs and Glutes | ☐ Full Body

I feel: 😊 😐 🙁

Sleep quantity and quality: _____

Workout notes: _____

FRIDAY

□□□□□□□□ 🍎🍎 🌿🌿🌿🌿

☐ Core and Abs | ☐ Legs and Glutes | ☐ Full Body

I feel: 😊 😐 🙁

Sleep quantity and quality: _____

Workout notes: _____

SATURDAY

□□□□□□□□ 🍎🍎 🌿🌿🌿🌿

☐ Core and Abs | ☐ Legs and Glutes | ☐ Full Body

I feel: 😊 😐 🙁

Sleep quantity and quality: _____

Workout notes: _____

Weekly Fitness Journal

THIS WEEK'S GOALS:

1) _____

2) _____

3) _____

Check off daily intake of: Water 🥛 Fruit 🍎 Greens/veggies 🥬

SUNDAY

☐ Core and Abs | ☐ Legs and Glutes | ☐ Full Body

I feel: 😊 😐 🙁

Sleep quantity and quality: _____

Workout notes: _____

MONDAY

☐ Core and Abs | ☐ Legs and Glutes | ☐ Full Body

I feel: 😊 😐 🙁

Sleep quantity and quality: _____

Workout notes: _____

TUESDAY

☐ Core and Abs | ☐ Legs and Glutes | ☐ Full Body

I feel: 😊 😐 🙁

Sleep quantity and quality: _____

Workout notes: _____

WEDNESDAY

🥛🥛🥛🥛🥛🥛🥛🥛 🍎🍎 🌿🌿🌿🌿

☐ Core and Abs | ☐ Legs and Glutes | ☐ Full Body

I feel: 😊 😐 😟

Sleep quantity and quality: _____

Workout notes: _____

THURSDAY

🥛🥛🥛🥛🥛🥛🥛🥛 🍎🍎 🌿🌿🌿🌿

☐ Core and Abs | ☐ Legs and Glutes | ☐ Full Body

I feel: 😊 😐 😟

Sleep quantity and quality: _____

Workout notes: _____

FRIDAY

🥛🥛🥛🥛🥛🥛🥛🥛 🍎🍎 🌿🌿🌿🌿

☐ Core and Abs | ☐ Legs and Glutes | ☐ Full Body

I feel: 😊 😐 😟

Sleep quantity and quality: _____

Workout notes: _____

SATURDAY

🥛🥛🥛🥛🥛🥛🥛🥛 🍎🍎 🌿🌿🌿🌿

☐ Core and Abs | ☐ Legs and Glutes | ☐ Full Body

I feel: 😊 😐 😟

Sleep quantity and quality: _____

Workout notes: _____

Weekly Fitness Journal

THIS WEEK'S GOALS:

1) _____

2) _____

3) _____

Check off daily intake of: Water 🥛   Fruit 🍎   Greens/veggies 🌿

SUNDAY

☐ Core and Abs | ☐ Legs and Glutes | ☐ Full Body
I feel: 🙂 😐 🙁
Sleep quantity and quality: _____
Workout notes: _____

MONDAY

☐ Core and Abs | ☐ Legs and Glutes | ☐ Full Body
I feel: 🙂 😐 🙁
Sleep quantity and quality: _____
Workout notes: _____

TUESDAY

☐ Core and Abs | ☐ Legs and Glutes | ☐ Full Body
I feel: 🙂 😐 🙁
Sleep quantity and quality: _____
Workout notes: _____

WEDNESDAY

☐ Core and Abs | ☐ Legs and Glutes | ☐ Full Body

I feel: 😊 😐 😟

Sleep quantity and quality: _____

Workout notes: _____

THURSDAY

☐ Core and Abs | ☐ Legs and Glutes | ☐ Full Body

I feel: 😊 😐 😟

Sleep quantity and quality: _____

Workout notes: _____

FRIDAY

☐ Core and Abs | ☐ Legs and Glutes | ☐ Full Body

I feel: 😊 😐 😟

Sleep quantity and quality: _____

Workout notes: _____

SATURDAY

☐ Core and Abs | ☐ Legs and Glutes | ☐ Full Body

I feel: 😊 😐 😟

Sleep quantity and quality: _____

Workout notes: _____

Weekly Fitness Journal

THIS WEEK'S GOALS:

1) _____

2) _____

3) _____

Check off daily intake of: Water 🥛 Fruit 🍎 Greens/veggies 🌿

SUNDAY

🥛🥛🥛🥛🥛🥛🥛🥛 🍎🍎 🌿🌿🌿🌿

☐ Core and Abs | ☐ Legs and Glutes | ☐ Full Body

I feel: 😊 😐 ☹️

Sleep quantity and quality: _____

Workout notes: _____

MONDAY

🥛🥛🥛🥛🥛🥛🥛🥛 🍎🍎 🌿🌿🌿🌿

☐ Core and Abs | ☐ Legs and Glutes | ☐ Full Body

I feel: 😊 😐 ☹️

Sleep quantity and quality: _____

Workout notes: _____

TUESDAY

🥛🥛🥛🥛🥛🥛🥛🥛 🍎🍎 🌿🌿🌿🌿

☐ Core and Abs | ☐ Legs and Glutes | ☐ Full Body

I feel: 😊 😐 ☹️

Sleep quantity and quality: _____

Workout notes: _____

WEDNESDAY

☐ Core and Abs | ☐ Legs and Glutes | ☐ Full Body

I feel: 😊 😐 ☹️

Sleep quantity and quality: _____

Workout notes: _____

THURSDAY

☐ Core and Abs | ☐ Legs and Glutes | ☐ Full Body

I feel: 😊 😐 ☹️

Sleep quantity and quality: _____

Workout notes: _____

FRIDAY

☐ Core and Abs | ☐ Legs and Glutes | ☐ Full Body

I feel: 😊 😐 ☹️

Sleep quantity and quality: _____

Workout notes: _____

SATURDAY

☐ Core and Abs | ☐ Legs and Glutes | ☐ Full Body

I feel: 😊 😐 ☹️

Sleep quantity and quality: _____

Workout notes: _____

Weekly Fitness Journal

THIS WEEK'S GOALS:

1) _____

2) _____

3) _____

Check off daily intake of: Water 🥛 Fruit 🍎 Greens/veggies 🌿

SUNDAY

🥛🥛🥛🥛🥛🥛🥛🥛 🍎🍎 🌿🌿🌿🌿

☐ Core and Abs | ☐ Legs and Glutes | ☐ Full Body

I feel: 😊 😐 🙁

Sleep quantity and quality: _____

Workout notes: _____

MONDAY

🥛🥛🥛🥛🥛🥛🥛🥛 🍎🍎 🌿🌿🌿🌿

☐ Core and Abs | ☐ Legs and Glutes | ☐ Full Body

I feel: 😊 😐 🙁

Sleep quantity and quality: _____

Workout notes: _____

TUESDAY

🥛🥛🥛🥛🥛🥛🥛🥛 🍎🍎 🌿🌿🌿🌿

☐ Core and Abs | ☐ Legs and Glutes | ☐ Full Body

I feel: 😊 😐 🙁

Sleep quantity and quality: _____

Workout notes: _____

WEDNESDAY

□ Core and Abs | □ Legs and Glutes | □ Full Body

I feel: 😊 😐 🙁

Sleep quantity and quality: _____

Workout notes: _____

THURSDAY

□ Core and Abs | □ Legs and Glutes | □ Full Body

I feel: 😊 😐 🙁

Sleep quantity and quality: _____

Workout notes: _____

FRIDAY

□ Core and Abs | □ Legs and Glutes | □ Full Body

I feel: 😊 😐 🙁

Sleep quantity and quality: _____

Workout notes: _____

SATURDAY

□ Core and Abs | □ Legs and Glutes | □ Full Body

I feel: 😊 😐 🙁

Sleep quantity and quality: _____

Workout notes: _____

Weekly Fitness Journal

THIS WEEK'S GOALS:

1) _____

2) _____

3) _____

Check off daily intake of: Water 🥛 Fruit 🍎 Greens/veggies 🌿

SUNDAY

🥛🥛🥛🥛🥛🥛🥛🥛 🍎🍎 🌿🌿🌿🌿

☐ Core and Abs | ☐ Legs and Glutes | ☐ Full Body

I feel: 🙂 😐 🙁

Sleep quantity and quality: _____

Workout notes: _____

MONDAY

🥛🥛🥛🥛🥛🥛🥛🥛 🍎🍎 🌿🌿🌿🌿

☐ Core and Abs | ☐ Legs and Glutes | ☐ Full Body

I feel: 🙂 😐 🙁

Sleep quantity and quality: _____

Workout notes: _____

TUESDAY

🥛🥛🥛🥛🥛🥛🥛🥛 🍎🍎 🌿🌿🌿🌿

☐ Core and Abs | ☐ Legs and Glutes | ☐ Full Body

I feel: 🙂 😐 🙁

Sleep quantity and quality: _____

Workout notes: _____

WEDNESDAY

☐ Core and Abs | ☐ Legs and Glutes | ☐ Full Body

I feel: 😊 😐 ☹️

Sleep quantity and quality: _____

Workout notes: _____

THURSDAY

☐ Core and Abs | ☐ Legs and Glutes | ☐ Full Body

I feel: 😊 😐 ☹️

Sleep quantity and quality: _____

Workout notes: _____

FRIDAY

☐ Core and Abs | ☐ Legs and Glutes | ☐ Full Body

I feel: 😊 😐 ☹️

Sleep quantity and quality: _____

Workout notes: _____

SATURDAY

☐ Core and Abs | ☐ Legs and Glutes | ☐ Full Body

I feel: 😊 😐 ☹️

Sleep quantity and quality: _____

Workout notes: _____

Weekly Fitness Journal

THIS WEEK'S GOALS:

1) _____

2) _____

3) _____

Check off daily intake of: Water 🥛 Fruit 🍎 Greens/veggies 🌿

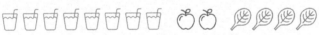

SUNDAY

☐ Core and Abs | ☐ Legs and Glutes | ☐ Full Body

I feel: 🙂 😐 🙁

Sleep quantity and quality: _____

Workout notes: _____

MONDAY

☐ Core and Abs | ☐ Legs and Glutes | ☐ Full Body

I feel: 🙂 😐 🙁

Sleep quantity and quality: _____

Workout notes: _____

TUESDAY

☐ Core and Abs | ☐ Legs and Glutes | ☐ Full Body

I feel: 🙂 😐 🙁

Sleep quantity and quality: _____

Workout notes: _____

WEDNESDAY

☐ Core and Abs | ☐ Legs and Glutes | ☐ Full Body

I feel: 😊 😐 ☹

Sleep quantity and quality: _____

Workout notes: _____

THURSDAY

☐ Core and Abs | ☐ Legs and Glutes | ☐ Full Body

I feel: 😊 😐 ☹

Sleep quantity and quality: _____

Workout notes: _____

FRIDAY

☐ Core and Abs | ☐ Legs and Glutes | ☐ Full Body

I feel: 😊 😐 ☹

Sleep quantity and quality: _____

Workout notes: _____

SATURDAY

☐ Core and Abs | ☐ Legs and Glutes | ☐ Full Body

I feel: 😊 😐 ☹

Sleep quantity and quality: _____

Workout notes: _____

Weekly Fitness Journal

THIS WEEK'S GOALS:

1) _____

2) _____

3) _____

Check off daily intake of: Water 🥛 Fruit 🍎 Greens/veggies 🥬

SUNDAY

☐ Core and Abs | ☐ Legs and Glutes | ☐ Full Body

I feel: 🙂 😐 🙁

Sleep quantity and quality: _____

Workout notes: _____

MONDAY

☐ Core and Abs | ☐ Legs and Glutes | ☐ Full Body

I feel: 🙂 😐 🙁

Sleep quantity and quality: _____

Workout notes: _____

TUESDAY

☐ Core and Abs | ☐ Legs and Glutes | ☐ Full Body

I feel: 🙂 😐 🙁

Sleep quantity and quality: _____

Workout notes: _____

WEDNESDAY

☐ Core and Abs | ☐ Legs and Glutes | ☐ Full Body

I feel: 😊 😐 ☹

Sleep quantity and quality: _____

Workout notes: _____

THURSDAY

☐ Core and Abs | ☐ Legs and Glutes | ☐ Full Body

I feel: 😊 😐 ☹

Sleep quantity and quality: _____

Workout notes: _____

FRIDAY

☐ Core and Abs | ☐ Legs and Glutes | ☐ Full Body

I feel: 😊 😐 ☹

Sleep quantity and quality: _____

Workout notes: _____

SATURDAY

☐ Core and Abs | ☐ Legs and Glutes | ☐ Full Body

I feel: 😊 😐 ☹

Sleep quantity and quality: _____

Workout notes: _____

Weekly Fitness Journal

THIS WEEK'S GOALS:

1) _____

2) _____

3) _____

Check off daily intake of: Water 🥛 Fruit 🍎 Greens/veggies 🌿

SUNDAY

🥛🥛🥛🥛🥛🥛🥛🥛 🍎🍎 🌿🌿🌿🌿

☐ Core and Abs | ☐ Legs and Glutes | ☐ Full Body

I feel: 🙂 😐 🙁

Sleep quantity and quality: _____

Workout notes: _____

MONDAY

🥛🥛🥛🥛🥛🥛🥛🥛 🍎🍎 🌿🌿🌿🌿

☐ Core and Abs | ☐ Legs and Glutes | ☐ Full Body

I feel: 🙂 😐 🙁

Sleep quantity and quality: _____

Workout notes: _____

TUESDAY

🥛🥛🥛🥛🥛🥛🥛🥛 🍎🍎 🌿🌿🌿🌿

☐ Core and Abs | ☐ Legs and Glutes | ☐ Full Body

I feel: 🙂 😐 🙁

Sleep quantity and quality: _____

Workout notes: _____

WEDNESDAY

☐ Core and Abs | ☐ Legs and Glutes | ☐ Full Body

I feel: 😊 😐 🙁

Sleep quantity and quality: _____

Workout notes: _____

THURSDAY

☐ Core and Abs | ☐ Legs and Glutes | ☐ Full Body

I feel: 😊 😐 🙁

Sleep quantity and quality: _____

Workout notes: _____

FRIDAY

☐ Core and Abs | ☐ Legs and Glutes | ☐ Full Body

I feel: 😊 😐 🙁

Sleep quantity and quality: _____

Workout notes: _____

SATURDAY

☐ Core and Abs | ☐ Legs and Glutes | ☐ Full Body

I feel: 😊 😐 🙁

Sleep quantity and quality: _____

Workout notes: _____

Weekly Fitness Journal

THIS WEEK'S GOALS:

1) _____

2) _____

3) _____

Check off daily intake of: Water 🥛 Fruit 🍎 Greens/veggies 🌿

SUNDAY

☐ Core and Abs | ☐ Legs and Glutes | ☐ Full Body

I feel: 😊 😐 ☹️

Sleep quantity and quality: _____

Workout notes: _____

MONDAY

☐ Core and Abs | ☐ Legs and Glutes | ☐ Full Body

I feel: 😊 😐 ☹️

Sleep quantity and quality: _____

Workout notes: _____

TUESDAY

☐ Core and Abs | ☐ Legs and Glutes | ☐ Full Body

I feel: 😊 😐 ☹️

Sleep quantity and quality: _____

Workout notes: _____

WEDNESDAY

☐ Core and Abs | ☐ Legs and Glutes | ☐ Full Body

I feel: 🙂 😐 🙁

Sleep quantity and quality: _____

Workout notes: _____

THURSDAY

☐ Core and Abs | ☐ Legs and Glutes | ☐ Full Body

I feel: 🙂 😐 🙁

Sleep quantity and quality: _____

Workout notes: _____

FRIDAY

☐ Core and Abs | ☐ Legs and Glutes | ☐ Full Body

I feel: 🙂 😐 🙁

Sleep quantity and quality: _____

Workout notes: _____

SATURDAY

☐ Core and Abs | ☐ Legs and Glutes | ☐ Full Body

I feel: 🙂 😐 🙁

Sleep quantity and quality: _____

Workout notes: _____

Weekly Fitness Journal

THIS WEEK'S GOALS:

1) _____

2) _____

3) _____

Check off daily intake of: Water 🥛 Fruit 🍎 Greens/veggies 🌿

SUNDAY

🥛🥛🥛🥛🥛🥛🥛🥛 🍎🍎 🌿🌿🌿🌿

☐ Core and Abs | ☐ Legs and Glutes | ☐ Full Body

I feel: 🙂 😐 🙁

Sleep quantity and quality: _____

Workout notes: _____

MONDAY

🥛🥛🥛🥛🥛🥛🥛🥛 🍎🍎 🌿🌿🌿🌿

☐ Core and Abs | ☐ Legs and Glutes | ☐ Full Body

I feel: 🙂 😐 🙁

Sleep quantity and quality: _____

Workout notes: _____

TUESDAY

🥛🥛🥛🥛🥛🥛🥛🥛 🍎🍎 🌿🌿🌿🌿

☐ Core and Abs | ☐ Legs and Glutes | ☐ Full Body

I feel: 🙂 😐 🙁

Sleep quantity and quality: _____

Workout notes: _____

WEDNESDAY

☐ Core and Abs | ☐ Legs and Glutes | ☐ Full Body

I feel: 😊 😐 ☹️

Sleep quantity and quality: _____

Workout notes: _____

THURSDAY

☐ Core and Abs | ☐ Legs and Glutes | ☐ Full Body

I feel: 😊 😐 ☹️

Sleep quantity and quality: _____

Workout notes: _____

FRIDAY

☐ Core and Abs | ☐ Legs and Glutes | ☐ Full Body

I feel: 😊 😐 ☹️

Sleep quantity and quality: _____

Workout notes: _____

SATURDAY

☐ Core and Abs | ☐ Legs and Glutes | ☐ Full Body

I feel: 😊 😐 ☹️

Sleep quantity and quality: _____

Workout notes: _____

Weekly Fitness Journal

THIS WEEK'S GOALS:

1) _____

2) _____

3) _____

Check off daily intake of: Water 🥛 Fruit 🍎 Greens/veggies 🥬

SUNDAY

☐ Core and Abs | ☐ Legs and Glutes | ☐ Full Body

I feel: 😊 😐 🙁

Sleep quantity and quality: _____

Workout notes: _____

MONDAY

☐ Core and Abs | ☐ Legs and Glutes | ☐ Full Body

I feel: 😊 😐 🙁

Sleep quantity and quality: _____

Workout notes: _____

TUESDAY

☐ Core and Abs | ☐ Legs and Glutes | ☐ Full Body

I feel: 😊 😐 🙁

Sleep quantity and quality: _____

Workout notes: _____

WEDNESDAY

🥛🥛🥛🥛🥛🥛🥛🥛 🍎🍎 🥬🥬🥬🥬

☐ Core and Abs | ☐ Legs and Glutes | ☐ Full Body

I feel: 😊 😐 😟

Sleep quantity and quality: _____

Workout notes: _____

THURSDAY

🥛🥛🥛🥛🥛🥛🥛🥛 🍎🍎 🥬🥬🥬🥬

☐ Core and Abs | ☐ Legs and Glutes | ☐ Full Body

I feel: 😊 😐 😟

Sleep quantity and quality: _____

Workout notes: _____

FRIDAY

🥛🥛🥛🥛🥛🥛🥛🥛 🍎🍎 🥬🥬🥬🥬

☐ Core and Abs | ☐ Legs and Glutes | ☐ Full Body

I feel: 😊 😐 😟

Sleep quantity and quality: _____

Workout notes: _____

SATURDAY

🥛🥛🥛🥛🥛🥛🥛🥛 🍎🍎 🥬🥬🥬🥬

☐ Core and Abs | ☐ Legs and Glutes | ☐ Full Body

I feel: 😊 😐 😟

Sleep quantity and quality: _____

Workout notes: _____

Weekly Fitness Journal

THIS WEEK'S GOALS:

1) _____

2) _____

3) _____

Check off daily intake of: Water 🥛 Fruit 🍎 Greens/veggies 🌿

SUNDAY

🥛🥛🥛🥛🥛🥛🥛🥛 🍎🍎 🌿🌿🌿🌿

☐ Core and Abs | ☐ Legs and Glutes | ☐ Full Body

I feel: 😊 😐 🙁

Sleep quantity and quality: _____

Workout notes: _____

MONDAY

🥛🥛🥛🥛🥛🥛🥛🥛 🍎🍎 🌿🌿🌿🌿

☐ Core and Abs | ☐ Legs and Glutes | ☐ Full Body

I feel: 😊 😐 🙁

Sleep quantity and quality: _____

Workout notes: _____

TUESDAY

🥛🥛🥛🥛🥛🥛🥛🥛 🍎🍎 🌿🌿🌿🌿

☐ Core and Abs | ☐ Legs and Glutes | ☐ Full Body

I feel: 😊 😐 🙁

Sleep quantity and quality: _____

Workout notes: _____

WEDNESDAY

🥛🥛🥛🥛🥛🥛🥛🥛 🍎🍎 🍃🍃🍃🍃

☐ Core and Abs | ☐ Legs and Glutes | ☐ Full Body

I feel: 😊 😐 ☹️

Sleep quantity and quality: _____

Workout notes: _____

THURSDAY

🥛🥛🥛🥛🥛🥛🥛🥛 🍎🍎 🍃🍃🍃🍃

☐ Core and Abs | ☐ Legs and Glutes | ☐ Full Body

I feel: 😊 😐 ☹️

Sleep quantity and quality: _____

Workout notes: _____

FRIDAY

🥛🥛🥛🥛🥛🥛🥛🥛 🍎🍎 🍃🍃🍃🍃

☐ Core and Abs | ☐ Legs and Glutes | ☐ Full Body

I feel: 😊 😐 ☹️

Sleep quantity and quality: _____

Workout notes: _____

SATURDAY

🥛🥛🥛🥛🥛🥛🥛🥛 🍎🍎 🍃🍃🍃🍃

☐ Core and Abs | ☐ Legs and Glutes | ☐ Full Body

I feel: 😊 😐 ☹️

Sleep quantity and quality: _____

Workout notes: _____

Weekly Fitness Journal

THIS WEEK'S GOALS:

1) _____

2) _____

3) _____

Check off daily intake of: Water 🥛 Fruit 🍎 Greens/veggies 🌿

SUNDAY

🥛🥛🥛🥛🥛🥛🥛🥛 🍎🍎 🌿🌿🌿🌿

☐ Core and Abs | ☐ Legs and Glutes | ☐ Full Body

I feel: 😊 😐 🙁

Sleep quantity and quality: _____

Workout notes: _____

MONDAY

🥛🥛🥛🥛🥛🥛🥛🥛 🍎🍎 🌿🌿🌿🌿

☐ Core and Abs | ☐ Legs and Glutes | ☐ Full Body

I feel: 😊 😐 🙁

Sleep quantity and quality: _____

Workout notes: _____

TUESDAY

🥛🥛🥛🥛🥛🥛🥛🥛 🍎🍎 🌿🌿🌿🌿

☐ Core and Abs | ☐ Legs and Glutes | ☐ Full Body

I feel: 😊 😐 🙁

Sleep quantity and quality: _____

Workout notes: _____

WEDNESDAY

☐ Core and Abs | ☐ Legs and Glutes | ☐ Full Body
I feel: 🙂 😐 🙁
Sleep quantity and quality: _____
Workout notes: _____

THURSDAY

☐ Core and Abs | ☐ Legs and Glutes | ☐ Full Body
I feel: 🙂 😐 🙁
Sleep quantity and quality: _____
Workout notes: _____

FRIDAY

☐ Core and Abs | ☐ Legs and Glutes | ☐ Full Body
I feel: 🙂 😐 🙁
Sleep quantity and quality: _____
Workout notes: _____

SATURDAY

☐ Core and Abs | ☐ Legs and Glutes | ☐ Full Body
I feel: 🙂 😐 🙁
Sleep quantity and quality: _____
Workout notes: _____

Resources

These are some of my go-to resources for HIIT training, more workout options, or healthy meal ideas.

Eating Bird Food (blog), EatingBirdFood.com: You'll find lots of healthy meals and recipes here.

Fitness Blender (YouTube channel), YouTube.com/fitnessblender: This channel features many HIIT and low-impact workout options.

Fitnessista (blog); Fitnessista.com: This is my own website! I share lots of work-outs and recipe ideas, and my Fit Guide workouts are also available. I'd love to see you there!

HIIT Your Limit, by Len Kravitz, Ph.D. Apollo Publishers (2018): I've studied his work for years, and he's a HIIT genius.

Oh She Glows Everyday (blog), OhSheGlows.com: This site is all about vegan recipes.

Pinch of Yum (blog), PinchOfYum.com: This site has family-friendly meal ideas and great Instant Pot recipes.

References

Boutcher, Stephen H. "High-Intensity Intermittent Exercise and Fat Loss." *Journal of Obesity* 2011 (24 November 2010): Article ID 868305. doi.org/10.1155/2011/868305.

Diabetes.co.uk. "HIIT Fights Insulin Resistance in Women at Risk of Type 2 Diabetes." (August 2017). Diabetes.co.uk/news/2017/aug/hiit-fights -insulin-resistance-in-women-at-risk-of-type-2-diabetes-98446049.html.

Dupuy, Olivier, Wafa Douzi, Dimitri Theurot, Laurent Bosquet, and Benoit Dugué. "An Evidence-Based Approach for Choosing Post-Exercise Recovery Techniques to Reduce Markers of Muscle Damage, Soreness, Fatigue, and Inflammation: A Systematic Review with Meta-Analysis." *Frontiers in Physiology* 9 (26 April 2018). doi.org/10.3389/fphys.2018.00403.

Kravitz, Len. *HIIT Your Limit.* Apollo Publishers (2018).

Menz, Verena, Natalie Marterer, Sachin B. Amin, Martin Faulhaber, Alexander B. Hansen, and Justin S. Lawly. "Functional vs. Running Low-Volume High-Intensity Interval Training: Effects on VO$_2$max and Muscular Endurance." *Journal of Sports Science and Medicine* 18, no. 3 (September 2019): 497–504.

Penney, Stacey. "Hydration for Health and Performance." National Academy of Sports Medicine. January 17, 2014. blog.nasm.org/nutrition/hydration -health-performance.

Seldeen, Kenneth L., Ginger Lasky, Merced M. Leiker, Manhui Pang, Kirkwood E. Personius, and Bruce R. Troen. "High Intensity Interval Training Improves Physical Performance and Frailty in Aged Mice." *The Journals of Gerontology Series A Biological Sciences and Medical Sciences* 73, no. 4 (14 March 2018): 429–437. doi.org/10.1093/gerona/glx120.

Tabata, Izumi, Kouji Nishimura, Motoki Kouzaki, Yuusuke Hirai, Futoshi Ogita, Motohiko Miyachi, and Kaoru Yamamoto. "Effects of Moderate-Intensity Endurance and High-Intensity Intermittent Training on Anaerobic Capacity and VO$_2$max" *Medicine and Science in Sports and Exercise* 28, no. 10 (October 1996): 1327– 1330. doi.org/10.1097/00005768-199610000-00018.

Index

Acknowledgments

I'd love to thank the incredible team at Callisto for the opportunity to create this book, especially my editor, Nicky Montalvo. Thank you to my husband, Tom, for wrangling our two amazing girls while I spent extra time writing. Thank you to my blog family and readers of <u>Fitnessista.com</u>, my podcast audience, and those who have supported my endeavors over the years.

About the Author

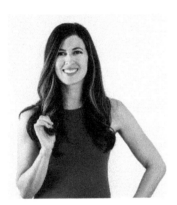

Gina Harney is the blogger behind the healthy lifestyle brand, *The Fitnessista*, which reaches millions of viewers all over the world. She's been featured in *Greatist*, *Forbes*, *Buzzfeed*, *Shape*, *Fitness Magazine*, and *Well + Good*. She's the author of *HIIT It!*, a contributor to the *WebMD Food and Fitness* blog, and the voice behind the *Healthy in Real Life* podcast. She lives in Tucson, Arizona, with her pilot husband, Tom, and two daughters, Olivia and Penelope.

CPSIA information can be obtained
at www.ICGtesting.com
Printed in the USA
JSHW012050200620
6266JS00006B/6